PC, M.D.

PC, M.D.

How Political Correctness Is Corrupting Medicine

SALLY SATEL, M.D.

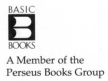

BASIC
BOOKS

A Member of the
Perseus Books Group

Published by Basic Books,
A Member of the Perseus Books Group

Designed by D. Gayle

Library of Congress Cataloging-in-Publication Data
Satel, Sally L.
    PC, M.D. : how political correctness is corrupting medicine /
Sally Satel.
        p.   cm.
    Includes bibliographical references and index.
    ISBN 0-465-07182-1 (cloth); ISBN 0-465-07183-X (pbk.)
    1. Medical care—United States—Miscellanea.   2. Political
correctness—United States.   3. Medical care—Social aspects—
United States.   4. Medicine—Social aspects—United States.
I. Title.

RA394 .S38   2000
362.1'0973—dc21

                                                        00-049813

02   03 / 10   9   8   7   6   5   4   3   2   1

To the Memory of
My Mother and Father

Contents

Acknowledgments

W HEN I WAS IN GRADUATE SCHOOL and later medical school, I had wonderful teachers. Their scholarship was first-rate, and they set high standards for all their students. When I had a serious illness in my twenties, I had superb physicians and nurses. Their priorities were in good order: patients before politics. And they treated all their patients alike, with compassion, integrity and skill. I wrote *PC, M.D.* out of gratitude, yes, but more acutely out of concern that the academic and clinical virtues I was taught are under threat.

I received financial and institutional support from a number of sources. I am most grateful to Elliott Abrams of the Ethics and Public Policy Center, Christopher DeMuth of the American Enterprise Institute, Elizabeth Lurie of the W. H. Brady Foundation and Antony Sullivan of the Earhart Foundation. The Center for Equal Opportunity helped defray research expenses, and the American Psychiatric Association library kindly made its resources available to me. In 1993 the Robert Wood Johnson Foundation gave me the unparalleled opportunity to learn lessons about the dynamics of policymaking through its congressional fellows program.

Many people generously read drafts and offered invaluable suggestions, in particular, Fred Sommers, Christina Hoff Sommers, Karlyn Bowman, Chris DeMuth, Christine Stolba, David Frum, Alan Swann and Tim Shah. Various chapters benefited enormously from the technical wisdom of Donal O'Mathuna, Seth Tanenbaum, William DeJong, Steve Southwick, Nicholas Eberstadt, Wallace Sampson, Robert Park, Allan Nissenson, S. Leonard Syme, David Sundwall, Jeffrey Geller, Andrew Kadar, Robert Gaston, Charlotte Hays, Linda DeGutis, Mary Ann Fralich, Edward Brandt, Roger Herdman, Lee Zwanziger, Patti Hausman, Theodore Marmor, Carl Roth, Barbara Liu, Steven Hyman, Steven Sharfstein, Ed Miller, David Murray, Robert Lichter, E. Fuller Torrey, Craig Nelson, Paul Leber, Jonathan Kerner, David Musto, Mark Kleiman and Harold Pollack. Neil Genzlinger and Leah Belsky were incisive readers, and Laura Merzig a gracious and energetic research assistant. Jo Ann Miller, executive editor of Basic Books, made suggestions with perfect pitch.

Finally, I thank my dear friends and colleagues whose warm encouragement sustained me throughout the project: the Sommerses, Barbara Ledeen, Sally Pipes, Mitchell Rosenthal, Neal Freeman, Ronald Docksai, Peter Collier, the late Robert Byck, Steve Bunney, David Gelernter, Deborah Fried and Rick Martinez. My fellow staff at the Oasis Clinic were exemplars of professional dedication.

Introduction

PC Medicine—Hazardous to Your Health

WHAT MAKES US SICK? Poison chemicals, viruses, smoking. These and hundreds of other things. But what about modern medicine itself?

More and more, social activists, scholars and even health professionals are telling us that the culture of medicine is to blame for many illnesses. No, they are not talking about health insurance woes, fifteen-minute office visits or medical mistakes. Here is what the critics are up to:

- A report in the *New England Journal of Medicine* claims that white men get the best treatment for heart disease. Other experts cite discrimination in the care of patients as a cause of differences in health between blacks and whites.

- Women's health advocates assert that the patriarchal medical establishment has kept women from participating as research subjects, depriving them of the benefits of medical breakthroughs.

- Former psychiatric patients, calling themselves "consumer-survivors," condemn the health care system for violating their human rights. They are on a crusade to "limit the powers of psychiatry by making consumers full partners in diagnosis and treatment."[1]

- Many nurses allege that they are oppressed by the male-dominated medical system and thus prevented from giving optimal service to patients.

- The 1998 Presidential Initiative on Race stated: "Research suggests that discrimination and racism create stress, leading to poorer health in minorities." Some public health experts use this "research" to scoff at physicians who urge people to take personal responsibility for protecting their own health.

The common theme here is the health profession's failure to make the connection between oppression—by society at large or by the medical establishment itself—and illness. It would be one thing if this were just a dry academic debate with no real-life consequences. But it isn't. The critics are beginning to fashion a world of politically correct medicine. I began to worry about this in 1995 when I learned that some of my fellow psychiatrists at a San Francisco hospital were grouping inpatients according to race and sexual orientation so that they could organize treatment around psychological needs that were supposedly peculiar to those groups.

This book shows what PC medicine looks like and how the very efforts to correct perceived problems are making some people sick, or sicker than they need to be. I begin in chapter 1 by examining the philosophy of PC medicine where it is most forcefully articulated, in the schools of public health. A former dean of the Harvard School of Public Health has described his institution as "a school of justice."[2] Indeed, it is true that society's sickest people tend also to be among its poorest and most disenfranchised, but many public health experts see their mission literally as attacking the conditions that lead to poverty and alienation in the first place. "The practice of public health," says Brown University's Sally Zierler, "is the process of redesigning society."[3] On the assumption that social conditions are the primary reason for ill health, she and her colleagues urge the redistribution of wealth to ensure the even distribution of health.

These political remedies may appeal to some—and to be sure, the relation between health and social status is not a trivial one—but what happens when a clinical enterprise like public health takes on the grandiose mission of "redesigning society"? For one thing, taking responsibility for one's own health comes to be virtually ignored. After all, if AIDS is a "biological expression of inequality," as Sally Zierler has put it, we can't hold people accountable if they place themselves at risk for contracting HIV, the virus that causes the disease. Indeed, we must understand that using a condom is hardly a priority for those who are "seeking sanctuary from racial hatred through sexual connection," as Zierler claims.[4] In this worldview, public health experts who want to fight the AIDS epidemic should be promoting social and economic justice, not self-care. Doctors like me, on the other hand, who expect their addicted patients to stop using drugs and to start using condoms—and if all else fails, to use clean needles—are accused of blaming the victim.

In the course of expanding the purview of public health to encompass the quest for social justice, the academic elite are warping the indispensable mission of their profession: the practical, here-and-now prevention of injury and disease. This is what we need and expect from public health. It is not equipped to fight widespread injustice and cannot squander on a utopian vision the energy and resources needed to prevent and combat the chronic diseases and disabilities from which Americans are suffering.

In PC medicine the quest for social justice can be mounted on any level, from academic campaigns to grassroots activism. Chapter 2 is about the reforms demanded by a group of people who call themselves "the last minority"—former psychiatric patients who once used or "consumed" mental health services and now say they have "survived" them. Claiming that the system has abused them, these "consumer-survivors" compare themselves to the civil rights warriors of the 1960s. Many revile medication and fight against public policies that make sure psychotic patients take antipsychotic drugs and, when necessary, hospitalize them against their will. Consumer-survivors want nothing less than control of the mental health system.

Are there problems with that system? As a psychiatrist, I say yes. But the consumer-survivors are making things worse for the severely mentally ill. Chances are that most readers have never heard of the consumer-survivor movement, but I have devoted a chapter to it because, as we shall see, it gets much of its funding from state and federal taxes—money siphoned away from treating mentally ill people who are genuinely sick, often help-less and sometimes dangerous. Aided by civil liberties lawyers, the con-sumer-survivors are acquiring real clout.

In Chapter 3 nurses are the ones who claim they are oppressed. To be sure, most nurses are dedicated to their jobs, suffer from serious staffing shortages and are worked to the bone. But a sizable fraction of them are disgruntled by what they perceive as a male-dominated system. Their misguided efforts to distance themselves from the medical "patri-archy" have led to a proliferation of fad therapies and a dumbing-down of nursing education—trends that can translate directly into botched diag-noses and care in medical centers and emergency rooms.

In Chapter 4 we again see women who claim mistreatment at the hands of a male-oriented society. These are the activists behind the mod-ern women's health movement, and as we will see, their complaints about receiving insufficient attention from the medical research and health care establishments have little basis in fact. It is not at all clear that the women's health advocates of today—unlike their feisty sisters from the 1960s and 1970s who brought us a welcome breath of fresh air in *Our Bodies, Ourselves*—can fairly point to sexism as a problem.

Chapter 5 takes us to South Carolina and the problems associated with crack-addicted women having babies. I tell the story of the quest for "social justice" for these women—that is, the lawyer-mounted campaign for their freedom to use cocaine during pregnancy—a crusade that has trampled on the best clinical interests of their newborns and of the moth-ers themselves. South Carolina was a flashpoint for this drama because it is the only state where a viable fetus is considered a person; as a result, when these mothers take drugs during the third trimester, they are tech-nically committing child abuse. As other states grapple with the rights of late-term fetuses, what happened in South Carolina will prove a riveting cautionary tale.

From South Carolina we return in Chapter 6 to Washington, D.C., where the federal government is trying to close the so-called health gap. While no one disputes the fact that minorities, especially black Americans, tend to be less healthy than whites, it is rash to ascribe this difference mainly to bias in the health care system or to doctors' subtle prejudice against minority patients. There are ample reasons for differences in health status—some easier to address than others—but the evidence does not support the charge of bias. The accusation is nonetheless being made by influential groups ranging from the U.S. Commission on Civil Rights to the Association of American Medical Colleges and by black leaders like the Reverend Al Sharpton. As if this rhetoric weren't divisive enough, some of the remedies being implemented are deeply worrisome.

The final chapter explores the strange new world of psychotherapy for victims. One aspect of this is "multicultural counseling," a practice strongly supported by the American Counseling Association. Multicultural counselors presume that nonwhite patients' personal difficulties largely stem from their efforts to adjust to a racist society. By urging patients to find only external sources for their discontent, multicultural counseling makes a mockery of self-exploration—the true purpose of therapy—and self-determination.

Most Americans are familiar with three eras of public health—the sanitation, biological and lifestyle eras. The first of these, the sanitation era, began in the mid-1800s and focused on the control of such contagious diseases as typhoid, tuberculosis and yellow fever. It ushered in developments like water purification, refuse disposal and extermination of disease-carrying pests. The late 1800s marked the start of the biological era, when the bacteria that cause specific diseases could actually be seen under the microscope. The first half of the twentieth century brought antibiotics, vaccines and pasteurization, and with them a series of rapid victories against devastating diseases such as polio, smallpox and diphtheria. The 1970s brought the lifestyle era, marked by campaigns against preventable injury and chronic illness. The surgeon general took the lead in urging Americans to stop smoking, reduce alcohol use, exercise more, eat less fat, use seat belts and wear bicycle helmets.

Over the last 150 years, millions of lives have been saved, improved, and extended by the public health efforts of these three eras. Through the honest application of science, education and a focus on personal responsibility, public health professionals have kept lethal elements from invading our bodies and helped us define the part we can play in preserving our own health.

So sweeping were the transformations in America's health during these eras that they are properly called revolutions. Now, at the turn of the twenty-first century, a fourth era, politically correct medicine, is emerging, powered by the idea that injustice produces disease and political empowerment is the cure. In stark contrast to the three revolutions that preceded it, the fourth "revolution" is counterfeit.

Though the activists appear to be waging "the good fight" for better health through social justice, their actions do not prevent disease, treat symptoms or perfect clinical methods. At best, they create distractions and waste money; at worst, they interfere with effective treatment. Although the activists themselves may end up feeling better, gratified to have taken part in the struggle for social justice, they undermine the Hippocratic ideal: the *patient* comes first.

PC medicine puts ideology before patients.

My goal is not to defend the status quo. There are many pressing problems, including how to deliver health care to everyone affordably. But it is critical to understand that injecting social justice into the mission of medicine diverts attention and resources from the effort to find ways of making everyone, regardless of race or sex, better off.

How did the activists—I call them "indoctrinologists," since their prescriptions for cure are ideology and social reform—manage to gain their foothold? One way is simple momentum. For several decades the universities, the law profession and the workplace have been under assault by people claiming oppression of one sort or another. It's almost surprising that medicine has been immune for so long. Another way is that the indoctrinologists' objectives play into a well-earned sense of guilt that hangs over the medical profession. Psychiatry, for example, has its skeletons in the closet, such as the dismal back wards of state mental hospitals. The reputation of the U.S. Public Health Service still smarts from the notorious Tuskegee Syphilis Study. Not too long ago women were expected to submit, without question, to radical mastectomies and hysterectomies simply because the (male) doctor recommended them.

Finally, PC medicine has flourished because too few people have been paying attention. While the nation has been preoccupied with head-line-grabbing subjects such as HMOs, Medicare coverage and the millions of uninsured Americans—all pressing issues indeed—the indoctrinolo-gists have swooped in under the radar. While it is improbable that this ac-tivist cohort of public health professors will ever spark public leaders and politicians into enacting the massive social reforms they dream of—in short, to equalize the health status of all Americans by redistributing wealth—their animating spirit is being felt in a number of clinical do-mains. Their efforts to administer PC medicine, as we will see, are gaining momentum, and their prescriptions will be hazardous to our health.

1

Public Health and the Quest for Social Justice

O NE OF THE MOST FAMOUS MOMENTS in public health took place in
1854 in the Golden Square area of London, which was reeling from
an epidemic of cholera. At the worst point five hundred people died over
a ten-day period. John Snow, a British physician who once attended to
Queen Victoria, got a map of London and marked the locations of the
homes of cholera victims. Using clever detective work, he pinpointed the
Broad Street pump as the source of the bacteria-contaminated water that
townspeople were carrying by bucketfuls into their homes.[1] Snow put the
pump on Broad Street out of commission by removing the handle, and
the cholera epidemic stopped virtually overnight.

Snow's triumphant removal of the Broad Street pump handle is the
stuff of medical legend. It harkens back to a simpler time when protection
from communicable diseases was the exclusive focus of the public health
profession. Its tasks were well defined—disease tracking and ensuring
food and water safety—and its victories dramatic. Today public health is
still very much concerned with infection control and epidemiology—the
study of diseases in populations—but over the last century its scope has
expanded to include activities such as monitoring air quality, administering public health services (such as vaccination programs and community-
based clinics) and preventing chronic conditions like asthma, diabetes and
heart disease. The effort to avert what were once called social diseases,

such as teen pregnancy, domestic violence and homelessness, is also within the orbit of public health.

Since many diseases and afflictions depend directly on living conditions, it was inevitable that public health would overlap with public policy. Indeed, the profession has always had a reformist spirit. In colonial times, for example, local governments passed sanitation laws and imposed fines for selling putrid meat or refusing to drain swamps. By the end of the 1800s some of those lessons had been forgotten. In fact, during the anti-tuberculosis campaigns in this country, reformers argued strenuously, and often to no avail, that fighting the disease went beyond personal hygiene: nutrition, housing and working conditions had to be improved as well.

In the early part of the twentieth century the "industrial hygiene" movement played an important role in condemning the working conditions of many laborers, such as coal miners and factory workers, and the needlessly hazardous conditions that resulted in severe injuries, lung disease and poisoning from mercury, radium and solvents. In doing so, these health professionals recalled the spirit of Rudolf Virchow, the nineteenth-century German biologist, physician and statesman who spoke eloquently about the effect of social conditions on fitness and health, even calling physicians the "natural attorneys of the poor."[2]

Documenting these phenomena and calling them to the attention of civic leaders is one thing. Some contemporary public health experts, however, have gone much further. As this chapter shows, a cadre of academics have put themselves in the business of condemning "competitive meritocracy," opposing the free market system, supporting affirmative action and derailing welfare reform—all in the name of health. Their rationale is simple: since health is inextricably tied to wealth and social position, we should try to equalize power in society. Hence the theme of the 1996 annual meeting of the American Public Health Association (APHA): "Empowering the Disadvantaged: Social Justice in Public Health."

No one would second-guess Snow's wisdom in disabling the Broad Street pump: it was causing the spread of cholera. Nor is there much dispute that public health professionals should monitor air quality or report infectious disease outbreaks or launch educational campaigns to discourage cigarette smoking, one of the most potent health risks. On the other hand, mobilizing against economic and social inequities to achieve the distant goal of better health is harder to justify. Yet, as we will see, many in the public health elite are putting more passion into the promotion of political doctrine than into direct efforts to improve health.

Postmodern Medicine

This new activism in public health is the outgrowth of "political correctness," which has deep philosophical roots in postmodernism. This popular social theory was first imported to the United States through the writings of Michel Foucault, the French social philosopher. Foucault condemned the "dominant culture" for imposing its values on society's powerless and disenfranchised members. In his view, postmodern man is a mere cog in the social machine. Although he may think in Enlightenment terms that he is rational and self-governing, according to Foucault he is a mere malleable product of culture.[3]

Certainly the social environments in which people grow up and live exert influence on their thoughts and actions. Yet postmodernists see the influence as so strong and pervasive that certain groups, such as minorities, are perpetual victims of the status quo. Many university professors have avidly embraced the postmodern doctrine. On college campuses it has become an ideological staple in the humanities, fine arts and social studies. Until recently, the applied sciences have been spared, but the postmodern trend is creeping into those domains as well: for example, the practitioners of PC medicine tell us that unless the dominant culture is toppled, we will never close the health gap between whites and blacks.

I am by no means the first to describe this worldview. The medical economist Robert G. Evans comments in his 1994 book *Why Are Some People Healthy and Others Not?* that, "for those on the left, health differentials are markers for social inequality and injustice more generally, and further evidence of the need to redistribute wealth and power, and restructure or overturn the existing social order."[4] That is exactly how Sally Zierler of Brown University's Department of Community Health sees AIDS—as "a biological expression of social inequality." During her lecture at the 1998 annual meeting of the American Public Health Association, I copied down her five recommendations for curbing the AIDS epidemic: limit the power of corporations, cap salaries of CEOs, eliminate corporate subsidies, prohibit corporate contributions to politicians and strengthen labor unions.[5]

Tuberculosis is another disease one might call a "biological expression" of disenfranchisement, since it primarily affects the poor, homeless and addicted. Yet it was New York City's hard-nosed decision in the early 1990s to require that everyone who needed medication take it daily, right in front of a health worker, that checked TB's spread. The workers' utopia envisioned by Zierler would have cured no one of TB, and it is a ludicrous anti-AIDS prescription. Why try to change society in the name of health when prevention strategies are already at hand?

Ironically, indoctrinologists who want nothing less than revolution in the name of health have been quick to condemn practical hygiene efforts as dangerous social intrusion. As Paul Starr notes in his sweeping history *The Social Transformation of American Medicine:* "The recent anti-Progressive historians, including both Marxists and liberals, tend to reclassify as social control events like the conquest of disease that were once appropriately regarded as historic achievements of human freedom. They remember the public health nurse who instructed mothers in infant hygiene as a kind of surreptitious agent of the police, insinuating bourgeois ideals into the authentic culture of the working class."[6] That the nurse may have taught mothers how to prevent their babies from dying, Starr says, we are now supposed to pass over as secondary and irrelevant.

Starr's observation exposes the hypocrisy of a movement that condemns the prevention of infections in infants as intolerable social control yet approves efforts to organize against capitalism and the meritocracy as pro-health. This paradox nicely captures the politicized culture of the new public health, a discipline whose practitioners consider themselves crusaders for social justice. As Brown's Sally Zierler herself told a journalist: "Those of us who were activists in the 1960s are now professors. This is a way of continuing the work [only] we are now working from the inside. In the 1950s we would have been blacklisted. We couldn't have had the agenda we have and be hired."[7]

That agenda is to bring about political change in the name of health. It is typically advanced in Marxist terms in which the world is a zero-sum game: "The good fortune of some [is seen] as the cause of ill fortune in others, whether in economic terms or in terms of health, love, or other benefits."[8] In other words, the good health of the well-off somehow depends on the poor being sick. As Paula Braverman, a physician with the medical school at the University of California at San Francisco, claims, "illness is caused by the power imbalance" inherent in a capitalist society. "Even if those living on the lowest rung of the social ladder had sufficient material resources," she said at a meeting of the American Public Health Association, "their health would still suffer because they are deprived relative to others." Accordingly, she urged the audience to "counteract the free market with social programs."[9]

Social Productionism

Starting in the early 1990s, a new academic enterprise called the "social production of disease" was born. Many scholars consider Richard G. Wilkinson, professor of social epidemiology at the University of Sussex, the father of "social production theory." That theory forms the basis of the study of social variables, among them classism, racism and sexism, that may contribute to disease.[10] Wilkinson's seminal 1992 article on the relationship between income and health was followed, as his colleagues put it, by "a virtual cascade of papers."[11] Social productionism posits two general pathways by which social disenfranchisement can lead to infirmity and shorter life expectancy. One is direct: through the stress of oppression. The other pathway is through material disadvantage and inferior access to health care, which take the greatest toll on the poor and on minorities, who are overrepresented among the poor.

It is well known that, on average, people who are further down on the socioeconomic ladder are less healthy and do not live as long as those above them. But the question is this: Is one's health totally at the mercy of social forces? Some public health experts come extremely close to saying yes. Rodney Clark of Wayne State University's Department of Psychology asserts that the emphasis on the role of personal responsibility in maintaining health constitutes a "subtler form of racism."[12] Richard S. Cooper, a physician with Loyola University Medical School in Chicago, is similarly pessimistic: "For all intents and purposes, black people in this society are imprisoned by institutional racism; this is the attribute of blackness which at bottom determines their health."[13] Hortensia Amaro of the Boston University School of Public Health says that "women's social status is a central feature of their risk for HIV."[14]

So powerful in fact are racism and sexism, claim Sally Zierler and her colleague Nancy Krieger, an epidemiologist at the Harvard School of Public Health, that they practically lead people to contract HIV from dirty needles and unprotected sex: "In response to daily assaults of racial prejudice and denial of dignity, women may turn to readily available mind altering substances for relief. . . . Seeking sanctuary from racial hatred through sexual connection as a way to enhance self-esteem . . . may offer rewards so compelling that condom use becomes less of a priority."[15]

According to academics like Krieger, Zierler, Cooper and Amaro, the fundamental prescription for HIV prevention is the eradication of power inequalities in our country. And as public health experts conduct more research on health and inequality, says Krieger, "a major implication for public health intervention [will] be policies promoting social and economic justice."[16]

No one disputes the fact that poor and disenfranchised people have fewer choices. At the very least, they cannot get medical care as easily. But is there no room for them to exercise personal responsibility over their health? The answer, according to Gladys H. Reynolds of the Centers for Disease Control (CDC), is no. To value self-care is to "bring issues of blame to our interpretations of sickness and health," she writes in the *Annals of Epidemiology*. Scolding her colleagues she says: "We the scientific community are no different from the public or the media: We bring everything we have been taught by our culture—our xenophobia, our homophobia, our racism, our sexism, our 'classism,' our tendency to 'otherize.'"[17]

Yet the notion that social forces are major determinants of health—that they are so overwhelming in fact that personal responsibility and self-care are reduced to quaint notions and middle-class values—is one of the most pernicious themes in PC medicine.

With the Centers for Disease Control (Reynolds's own institution) estimating that at least 50 percent of premature deaths are caused by diseases that have modifiable risk factors, it is downright reckless to diminish the vital role of personal behavior.[18] This is why regarding the patient, or the public, as a passive victim of malign social forces is a prescription for disaster.

Some of the greatest successes in public health have involved efforts to change personal behavior by educating the public about the risks of activities such as smoking, unhealthy eating and unprotected sex. As Richard Pasternack, director of preventive cardiology at Massachusetts General Hospital, says, "If you eliminate the factors that we know about, which are largely lifestyle issues—smoking, high blood pressure, high cholesterol, lack of exercise and diabetes—you can eliminate somewhere between 70 and 90 percent of disease in our population."[19]

But setting out to eliminate "racism" or "classism" in the name of health leaves a trail of problems. First, the upstream conditions targeted by indoctrinologists (such as income inequality) correlate with, but do not necessarily *cause*, ill health. Indeed, inferences about the causal pathway to a disease become less and less secure the further upstream one looks for the root cause—thus, there is no guarantee that the social revisions they seek would even improve health. Second, abstract proposals for attaining social justice have vast repercussions for other sectors of society. Unlike discrete vaccination programs and cancer screening campaigns, activist prescriptions for social restructuring are intended to go far beyond the confines of a health care agenda. Third, there is much we can do by ourselves to safeguard our own health through diet, exercise, safe sex and so on.

My faith in such choices and in our capacity to take advantage of them comes from my work as a staff psychiatrist in a methadone clinic in northeast Washington, D.C. Our patients come from the "other" Washington, where violence and crumbling housing projects are standard features of the landscape. Methadone, a long-acting heroin replacement, is a treatment of last resort for many addicts. Yet with the exception of a handful of mentally ill patients, it is the rare patient at our clinic who is clueless about how to get himself together. Most have been addicts on and off for so many years that there is little they don't know about what makes them vulnerable to relapse.

They know, for example, that boredom is one of their worst enemies—show me a bored substance abuser, and I'll show you someone who is seriously thinking about getting high. Users know that they have to stop associating with their drug-taking friends, and that it helps to spend time at Narcotics Anonymous meetings. They know that getting a job is more than just a way to make money. It keeps them busy, out of trouble, feeling productive and maybe even purposeful. Between help-wanted ads and training program announcements, my patients know how to get work. And most of them do.

Many of these men and women also know that they do best when external limits are placed on them. Those who are homeless may deliberately choose to stay at a local shelter that requires its residents to work or obtain a volunteer job. Such a shelter also helps them save some of their earnings and tests them for drugs on a weekly basis. A handful of patients talk about taking jobs, like truck-driving, that periodically drug-test. Patients who get a regular paycheck have their employer deposit it directly in their bank account so that they have no tempting cash on hand.

These are just some of the barriers that patients erect between themselves and their drugs. Not all of them want to take advantage of these techniques and the myriad other ways to protect themselves, but many patients choose to do so. Is it hard work? Most assuredly, but what can PC medicine offer them instead? Simply the demoralizing message that drug abusers truly don't have a choice or a chance—that is, until sexism and racism disappear and inequalities in wealth are abolished.

Advocacy in Academia—Part 1

The blurring of the boundaries between scholarship and political action is an ever-present risk in the classrooms of indoctrinologists. Mindy Thompson-Fullilove of the Columbia University School of Public Health exhorted her colleagues to "invent a new science that embodies human rights and civil rights essential to the health of human populations."[20]

Vincent Iacopino, a physician with the School of Public Health at the University of California at Berkeley, speaking at an American Public Health Association panel called "Putting Politics Back into Public Health Education," urged "merging the academy with advocacy."[21] He referred to the World Health Organization's oft-quoted definition of health—"a state of complete physical, mental and social well being, not merely the absence of disease or infirmity"—as justification for doing so.

Such an expansive definition of health probably explains why Deborah Prothrow-Stith of the Harvard School of Public Health gets so impatient with her colleagues: "At our worst, public health professionals can be self-righteous know-it-alls: emphasizing a violence prevention curriculum when people want and need jobs and economic development; focusing on lead paint removal when people are homeless; preaching abstinence when people are looking for someone to love them. . . . We sometimes just don't get it."[22]

Prothrow-Stith is right in naming homelessness, joblessness and insufficient love as causes of much suffering. But the job of public health is to prevent injury and illness in practical ways, including making the public aware of risks for accidents and disease and ways to minimize them. Incorporating abstract, broad social goals into schools of public health will only divert them from imparting their practical mission to students and society. "We have nearly converted the school of public health from an institution committed to developing the scientific bases for disease prevention into one of many arenas for advancing social justice, or some people's idea of social justice," writes Philip Cole and his colleagues of the public health school of the University of Alabama at Birmingham.[23]

Here is a sample of what Cole is referring to when he says that academic public health is increasingly devoted to "some people's idea of social justice." In her statement explaining why she should be elected to the APHA governing board, Mary Anne Mercer of the School of Public Health of the University of Washington at Seattle wrote that it was "painful to see the recent welfare 'reform' pass without an effective response from the public health community."[24] At the 1998 annual APHA meeting, Sally Zierler told audience members that their goal as public health professionals should be to overthrow the "competitive meritoc-racy." Why? Because, in her words, "unequal distribution of goods and ser-vices and property and profit means that deprived populations are less able to reduce [HIV infection] in their community."[25]

David G. Whiteis of Indiana-Purdue University, another social pro-duction researcher, has proclaimed that any public health policy that ig-nores "social justice is unworthy of the name." Whiteis literally calls for the designation of "poverty as a medical pathogen."[26] These matters make more appropriate subjects for politicians and activists, but indoctrinolo-gists like Whiteis insist that they lie squarely within their purview. After all, the argument goes, since the health status of a population is closely re-lated to wealth and social position, improving health depends on political empowerment.[27]

This reasoning is reflected in the broad definitions of public health that experts have put forth over the years. In 1920 C.-E. A. Winslow of the Yale School of Public Health proclaimed that, in addition to disease pre-vention and infection control, the profession should address the "devel-opment of the social machinery which will ensure to every individual . . . a standard of living adequate for the maintenance of health."[28] Others identified "decent housing, adequate income, freedom from war" as part of the public health mission.[29] Arguing for a redefinition of the field half a century later, Carl M. Shy of the University of North Carolina School of Public Health said it should be the "study of the distribution and social determinants of the health status of populations."[30]

Perhaps the most expansive outlook belongs to the former CDC di-rector William H. Foege of the Emory University School of Public Health in Atlanta. "Every problem is a public health problem," he said in 1993. "Our job in public health is to be indignant on behalf of everyone."[31] If Foege were correct, then it would indeed make sense to look to public health to solve all of society's problems. According to Lawrence Wallack of Portland State University and Lori Dorfman of the School of Public Health of the University of California at Berkeley, "The practice of public health is, to a large degree, the process of redesigning society. . . . It is more about closing the 'power gap' than the 'knowledge gap.'"[32] Academically speaking, postmodern medicine is best summed up by Harvey V. Fineberg, former dean of the Harvard School of Public Health: "A school of public health is like a school of justice."[33]

If it is the nature of a social movement to advance ever more expansive definitions of the problem over which it seeks to provoke public outrage, then public health, as envisioned by the academic elite, is very much a social movement. Moreover, it is a movement in which social reform and utopian vision often masquerade as health policy. This is a dramatic departure from the founding missions of the APHA and schools of public health.

In 1872 several physicians formed the American Public Health Association to promote the "sanitary sciences," and the following year the nation's first public health journal, *The Sanitarian,* made its appearance. The rapid progress in understanding the linkage between bacteria and contagious diseases hastened the development of new approaches to public health, so that by the turn of the nineteenth century it was becoming clear that specialized training was needed to perform the job of public health officer. In 1916 the School of Hygiene and Public Health was founded at Johns Hopkins University, and soon Harvard, Yale and Columbia had established such schools.

These institutions had a pragmatic focus on reducing disease and maintaining health. In pursuit of these aims, various disciplines came together in one academic setting: epidemiology to trace outbreaks of disease; vital statistics to measure birth and death rates; diagnostics for identifying contagious diseases; and bacteriology, toxicology, sanitation and food and water inspection. Public health was thus a discipline of inquiry and practice, not a sociopolitical movement. True, progressive city health departments in the mid-1800s, such as New York's, mounted actions against disease-promoting filth and congestion. And in the 1910s the APHA joined in the fight to influence government to ameliorate unhealthy factory conditions and eliminate decrepit and overcrowded housing. But these were practical reforms that addressed obvious and direct causes of illness and were driven by the recognition that dismal living and working conditions led to poor health. By contrast, the currents of political correctness now flowing through schools of public health and the APHA are generated not by local pragmatism to change real circumstances but by a global ideology to manipulate the way people think about disease and its remedies.

Advocacy in Academia—Part 2

So uncomfortable with social hierarchy are the PC academics that when they do field research (for example, comparing the effectiveness of two HIV prevention programs in a community), they bend over backward to deny the simple fact that the researchers generally know more than community leaders about how to do a study. "Socially and economically marginalized communities often have not had the power to name or define their own experience," states Barbara A. Israel of the University of Michigan School of Public Health. Her prescription: "All parties [should] participate as equal members and share control over all phases of the research process."[34] According to Ernest T. Stringer of Curtin University in Australia, the special training in inquiry should confer no special role in determining how the project should be designed. "All participants," he says, "[should] share the perquisites of privilege."[35]

This research style is known as "participatory research." Unfortunately, not all parties are qualified to participate. "Sometimes community leaders push a study question, but it is unanswerable because they don't know how to frame a hypothesis, operationalize variables and analyze data," according to a program director at the U.S. Department of Health and Human Services (HHS) Office of Maternal and Child Health who did not want to be named. "When you point this out, they can get very offended." M. Douglas Anglin, an addiction researcher at UCLA, experienced his own frustrations with local groups involved in a large-scale treatment project. "We spent hours educating members of these groups, one by one, on the limits of epidemiological research. They all loved the idea that they got a vote in designing the project, but we had to keep saying that you cannot do science by consensus if you want the work to be credible."[36]

But without collaboration, empowerment researchers say, they would not be able to achieve one of their major goals in attending to social inequalities through empowerment. How best to empower, however, is a subject of considerable debate. As Meredith Minkler and her colleague Nina Wallerstein of the University of New Mexico ask, "Can people in positions of dominance or privilege derived from culture, gender, race, or class empower others, or must people empower themselves? If empowerment includes the dimension of transferring power to others," they assert, "professionals may need to let go of their own power to make it more available to others."[37]

The implication of all this, Professor Cole of the University of Alabama points out, "is that nothing lies outside the realm of public health." Such mandates make schools of public health "all-inclusive, dilutes their resources and blur their focus."[38] As Donald E. Waite, professor emeritus of family medicine at Michigan State University College of Osteopathic Medicine, lamented to me, "The field has been co-opted by confused visionaries who are seeking what they view as a socialist utopia."[39] Indeed, epidemiology is being transformed from the study of disease in populations into a science for converting empirical findings—such as the demonstrated linkages between economic status and health—into a program of social action.[40]

It is a program whose barely concealed contempt for practical clinical achievement prompted the epidemiologist Kenneth Rothman and his colleagues to express their frustration: "It is remarkable that [we] are now chastised for our scientific accomplishments, which include such victories as the elaboration of the effects of tobacco smoking on many diseases, and the effect of folic acid on neural-tube defects. Countless other fragments of useful epidemiological knowledge have enabled many people to improve their health even if they could not avoid poverty and repression."[41]

Along with schools of public health, academic journals are also risking their reputation as neutral arbiters of science when they publish second-rate studies purporting to show that the haves are literally making the have-nots sick. Indeed, race and ethnicity research has been criticized by many scholars for "lack of rigour in conceptualization, terminology and interpretation," according to a survey by Trude Bennett and Raj Bhopal of the medical school at Newcastle-upon-Tyne.[42] With its strong emphasis on nonperformance criteria in admitting students to schools of public health—the American College of Epidemiology itself decries the "competitive meritocracy"—there is reason to worry about standards of scholarship.[43] The social production of disease seems well on its way to becoming the academic arm of the social justice movement in public health.

The gatekeepers of the scientific literature—the editors and peer reviewers—must be alert for weak science and for advocacy masquerading as scholarship. "These men and women are the safeguards against researchers indulging their ideologies," says David A. Savitz, professor of epidemiology at the University of North Carolina. "Mixing scientific and activist roles not only threatens the validity of our work, it sows doubt that our methods are even capable of rigor."[44] Alexander M. Walker of the Harvard School of Public Health acknowledges that public health researchers may have to draw on disciplines such as economics and sociology, but he rightly insists that "we need to [choose] theories that can be challenged and refuted."[45]

This is not to say that social production research is inevitably weak. Careful epidemiologists have produced first-rate analyses using social variables, such as accumulated wealth, educational level, church affiliation and community cohesion. The prevalence of venereal disease, for example, has been strongly linked to signs of neighborhood deterioration (such as garbage pileups, graffiti and abandoned cars) independent of the local poverty indices.[46] These researchers know that variables must be meticulously defined and measured.

A variable like "feeling discriminated against," however, is hard to measure and verify because it relies on a subject's inferences about the attitudes and intentions of another person (the potential discriminator). Not surprisingly, society can act as a Rorschach test pattern upon which individuals project their expectations and fears. For example, UCLA anthropologists found that many black customers interpreted the "relative restraint" of the demeanor of Korean American storekeepers as a sign of racism. Conversely, the storekeepers tended to interpret the "relatively personable involvement" of the black patrons as disrespectful.[47] How to separate such projections from true (intentional) racial discrimination? The National Institutes of Health (NIH) has recently taken on that demanding task. The agency is now awarding grants to study the relationship between health and "powerlessness," "discrimination," "racism" and "classism."[48] The epidemiologist David Savitz believes that this research could be useful, though he acknowledges how difficult it is to do properly. He urges peer reviewers and editors who judge the findings from such studies to maintain rigorous scientific standards.

Can Racism Make You Sick?

One avenue of social production research is the health effects of racial discrimination. Blood pressure is a good condition to evaluate in this context because it is easy to measure and responsive to stress. Moreover, high blood pressure, also called hypertension, is two to three times more likely to afflict black Americans than whites. Curiously, even when known risk factors such as diet and exercise are taken into account, blacks are still more likely to have high blood pressure. Several explanations have been posed—most often genetic predisposition or diet or a combination of the two—but the issue has continued to intrigue medical researchers.

In 1996 Nancy Krieger of the Harvard School of Public Health and her colleague, Stephen Sidney, a physician at a Kaiser Foundation Research Institute, claimed to have solved the white-black blood pressure puzzle: racism was the culprit. The stress of being a victim of racial bias, they say, could explain the higher levels of hypertension within the black population. Krieger and Sidney's study "Racial Discrimination and Blood Pressure" appeared in the *American Journal of Public Health,* and it made news instantly.[49]

"Study: Discrimination May Cause Hypertension in Blacks," declared the *Washington Post.*[50] National Public Radio broadcast a lengthy report in which one psychologist interviewed about the study said, "We now have concrete data showing that what society does to you affects your health."[51] The study has been widely cited, including in a 1998 report from President Clinton's Initiative on Race, which stated that "research suggests discrimination and racism create stress leading to poorer health [in minorities]."[52] Brent Staples, an editorial writer at the *New York Times*, wrote a column titled "Death by Discrimination? Of Prejudice and Heart Attacks."[53] Three years later Staples was still commenting on the study's findings, going so far as to remark that "the medical system has yet to list 'racism' as a cause of death [even though] some social scientists now see tension related to discrimination as a health hazard on par with smoking and a high fat diet."[54] It is not unreasonable to think that the stress of being a victim of discrimination could produce certain kinds of illnesses. After all, it is well established that many key physiological processes respond to psychological stress.[55] For example, our immune and hormonal systems and cardiovascular functioning can be affected by emotional states. And indeed, since the Krieger and Sidney article appeared in the fall of 1996, it has practically become a medical truism that racism doesn't just make its targets sick at heart but can make them physically ill as well.[56] As we will see, however, Krieger and Sidney's claim fails to pass scientific muster.

Blood Pressure and Racial Discrimination

What evidence do Nancy Krieger and Stephen Sidney put forth to support the conclusions they drew in their much-discussed 1996 article? They collected information on some forty-one hundred black and white men and women between the ages of twenty-five and thirty-seven who were questioned about their "experiences of racial discrimination and unfair treatment." The researchers asked, for example, whether the subjects had "ever been prevented from doing something (for example, getting a job, securing housing) or been hassled or made to feel inferior" because of their sex or race. They divided their subjects into three groups based on the number of times they reported having been victims of racial discrimination over their lifetimes: zero episodes, one or two episodes, or three or more episodes. Meanwhile, known risk factors for high blood pressure such as obesity and smoking were taken into account so that they would not skew the results. (The researchers, however, omitted salt intake, which is one of the major determinants of blood pressure levels, particularly in African Americans.)

The authors looked at individual blood pressure readings within the groups to see whether the levels correlated with the subjects' experiences of bias. They assumed that the incidents perceived by subjects as discriminatory produced an equal amount of distress in all of them; otherwise, there would be no reason to hypothesize a linear "dose-response" relationship between stress and blood pressure. But this questionable assumption became even more tenuous once the relationship between blood pressure levels and the reported episodes of discrimination was revealed.

Instead of showing a clear linkage between blood pressure and discrimination, the results were all over the map. Black working-class men and women who reported zero episodes of discrimination had higher blood pressure readings than those reporting one or more. Black professional women who reported one or two episodes of discrimination had lower blood pressure readings than those with none or with three or more. And black professional men with one or two episodes of discrimination had higher readings than those with none or with three or more.

Krieger and Sidney also asked subjects how they responded to being discriminated against: Did they "do nothing about it" or did they "talk to someone about it"? Again, the results were scattershot. The highest blood pressures were found among black working-class women who "did nothing," while black working-class men who "did nothing" had lower readings. Thus, in order to align the findings with the theory, Krieger and Sidney had to assume that the subjects underreported discrimination, either because their experiences of racism were "too painful to talk about" or because somehow the subjects felt they deserved to be treated unfairly because of their race, a process called internalized oppression. (The possibility that some subjects overreported episodes of discrimination was not entertained.)

Krieger and Sidney's assumptions about why subjects did or did not report certain experiences raise a red flag: conveniently, they can be used to explain away any finding that does not neatly fit the expected direction of the data. It is a standard rule of research that hypotheses must survive attempts to falsify them before they can be regarded as true (more precisely, as highly probable). In other words, Krieger and Sidney would have had to show that subjects reporting none or few episodes of discrimination did so for reasons other than that talking about such treatment was "too painful" or that they felt undeserving of respect. The catch is that internalized oppression, by its very nature, is not falsifiable. After all, how could Krieger and Sidney possibly know that their black subjects were in some way thinking they deserved mistreatment because of their race, especially when they were apparently unaware of those thoughts themselves? Nonetheless, the researchers confidently conclude, "Our results indicate that racial discrimination shapes patterns of blood pressure among the U.S. Black population."[57]

One more observation. The subjects studied by Krieger and Sidney were healthy men and women under age forty with normal blood pressures. In fact, the average blood pressure readings recorded—109/67 for black women and 115/72 for black men—would make any internist very happy, the ideal reading being 120/80. As these women and men age, it is likely that many will be diagnosed with hypertension (140/90 or higher). But those who develop the condition can count on this: if they faithfully take care of themselves, they will do a lot more for their health in a matter of weeks than could any campaign for social equality.

Research continues to show that self-management through medication and diet has considerable impact. According to the NIH "Hypertension Detection and Follow-up Study," the inverse relationship between education/socioeconomic status and elevated blood pressure disappears when patients take blood pressure medication.[58] Another large study called "Dietary Approaches to Stop Hypertension" (or DASH-Sodium) found that eating less salt can significantly reduce blood pressure.[59] Sometimes a low-salt diet can, by itself, correct high blood pressure, especially in black patients, who tend to have "salt-sensitive" hypertension more often than whites.[60] Thus, pharmaceutical and dietary changes can literally save lives *today* by averting stroke or heart attack.

The Redistribution of Health?

In addition to physiological changes supposedly engendered by the stress of oppression—the changes that Krieger and Sidney claimed to have found amid their scattered data—PC medicine emphasizes the relationship between health and wealth. To be sure, those higher up on the socioeconomic ladder, on average, enjoy better health than those below them. But does this mean that inhabitants of the lower rungs are necessarily doomed to illness and disability? Is it true, as David Whiteis of Indiana University says, that there is something about poverty itself that makes it a health problem? If so, would redistributing wealth (beyond simply extending health coverage) make poor people healthier?

A sizable number of public health experts think so and advocate as much in a 1999 collection of essays called *The Society and Population Health Reader: Income Inequality and Health.* "The higher health achievement of egalitarian societies makes a persuasive case for the redistribution of income," claim the *Reader*'s editors, who are from the Harvard School of Public Health and the University of Sussex, England.[61] Clearly, this is a complicated and politically delicate issue. With that in mind, let us explore the basic interactions between health and wealth.

In general, the wealthier one is, the healthier one is. In London during the Black Plague in the 1660s, the wealthy had the means to flee the infested inner cities; they also benefited from better nutrition and sanitation, which made them more resistant to bubonic plague and more likely to survive if infected. In the modern era, too, wealth gives people access to better health care, better nutrition and better living and occupational conditions.

Conversely, people who are healthy are more likely to hold jobs and to work competitively, activities that help them advance their socioeconomic position and, in turn, protect their health. Sociologists call this the healthy worker effect. The pattern is especially obvious among the elderly members of minority groups. Because of poorer health histories, they are much more likely to lose functional ability than are whites and so are unable to generate income in their senior years.[62]

The overall probability of dying between the ages of twenty-five and sixty-four has been declining since 1960, but poor and poorly educated people still die younger.[63] This phenomenon is related to a host of factors over which people have minimal day-to-day control. For example, low-paying jobs tend to have less flexible hours, making it difficult for the worker to fit in doctors' appointments or take the day off when they have the flu. Simply finding a reliable baby-sitter in order to take two city buses to the doctor can be a major task. Poorer people cannot afford to buy bigger, safer cars, and they are more likely to be the victims of violent crime. They generally know less about how to stay healthy. Social service bureaucracies can be intimidating, waiting lists stalled and scheduling inconvenient. (I once tried to refer a patient to a free clinic in Baltimore, but I was permitted to call the intake counselor only between seven and eight o'clock in the morning on Wednesdays.)

When these forces influence health and access to care, it makes sense to say that "social class gets into the body," in the words of Nancy Moss of the Pacific Institute for Women's Health.[64] I think about my patients whose children have asthma. This lung condition has been on the rise since the 1980s and now afflicts about five million children. Black children are four to six times as likely to die from it as white children.[65] One important trigger for asthma, especially among inner-city kids, is the mundane cockroach.[66] Tiny parts of the insects' bodies are shed and inhaled, causing allergic reactions that constrict small airway passages in the lungs. My patients (mainly single mothers) may keep a clean apartment, but there is little they can do about their neighbors' housekeeping habits. The city may eventually get around to fumigating, but the roaches (and the rodents and the dust mites) come back because the neighbors don't change their habits.

Social class got "into the body" of the son of one of my patients who was burned out of her apartment house by a neighbor who fell asleep with a cigarette. She had no fire insurance, and her only local relative, a sister, with whom she fleetingly considered staying, sometimes smoked crack and had an alcoholic boyfriend. So the mother and son spent weeks in a damp shelter until the asthmatic child developed pneumonia and had to be hospitalized. In these situations I am more of a social worker than a physician as I try to help people navigate the District of Columbia's impossibly byzantine social services maze.

Then, of course, there are the obvious issues of access to care. Low-wage workers and minorities are less likely to have employer-based health insurance than are better-paid employees.[67] Not having a regular source of care is a big obstacle to receiving timely care and maintaining a familiar relationship with a doctor. Even when they are enrolled in managed care, minorities are more likely to pay the price when managed care plans weed out doctors with caseloads weighted with Medicaid-insured patients or sicker—and thus more costly—patients. Patients themselves can be excluded from plans if their care is too expensive, and older patients are penalized when nursing homes limit the number of Medicaid recipients they accept or when home health workers refuse to make visits in dangerous neighborhoods.[68]

Finally, simply having insurance can itself be a proxy for social and attitudinal factors that influence health. For example, a 1993 study of thousands of New Jersey women with invasive breast cancer found that women who were not privately insured received the diagnosis later and died sooner after diagnosis than those with private insurance.[69] Obviously, private insurance means better access to care, but coverage of services is not always enough. In fact, the New Jersey women whose mammogram costs were covered by public insurance did as poorly as those with no coverage at all. Why? In large part because women who live on the lower rungs of the socioeconomic ladder are more likely to deny cancer symptoms, to distrust the medical system and to fail to perform self-examination. Some are not aware that public insurance will pay for screening services. These are all possible explanations for higher mortality among poor women.

Putting Correlation in Perspective

Bruce G. Link of the Columbia University School of Public Health and Jo C. Phelan, a sociologist at UCLA, urge us to view socioeconomic status as a "fundamental cause" of disease. "If we truly wish to reduce inequalities in health," they advise in the *American Journal of Public Health*, "we must address the social inequalities that so reliably produce them."[70] But just how reliably do social conditions actually cause disease? It is crucial to realize that many "determinants" of disease are really *correlates* of disease, not necessarily direct causes of it. Social inequalities are associated with the habits and limited opportunities that often lead to poorer health, but they do not literally produce the sedentary lifestyle, obesity and risky behavior that typically underlie many of the differences in health status between the less wealthy and the better-off.

Another point of confusion is the assumption that what is true about a population's health is also necessarily true about an individual from that population—an unfounded conclusion that sociologists call the ecological fallacy. True, it may be a statistical fact that one out of every three young black inner-city men ends up involved with the criminal justice system by age twenty, but this need not be the future for any particular young black man. Even a low level of education does not inevitably lead to poor prospects. A high school dropout need not succumb to his statistical fate; he *can* get a GED, take college courses, postpone having children until married, exercise regularly, refrain from smoking and drinking and thereby greatly improve his financial and medical fortunes.

There is no denying the pressures on him—one of the most malignant, in my view, is the pressure exerted by his own peers to fail in school—but the institutions that will bolster him are neither built nor maintained by the public health profession. It is civil society and its members—qualified teachers unafraid to discipline, attentive parents, interested neighbors and others—that are crucial to this young man.

Because public health focuses on populations, not on individuals, its research properly concerns the relationship between particular variables (for example, pollution, income, diet) and the health status of groups. Even so, it is striking that indoctrinologists consistently home in on aspects of these relationships that fit a particular political orientation. For example, noting that wealth and health correlate, some public health experts condemn capitalism and decry efforts to roll back entitlement programs and racial preferences in college admissions. However, if they must be social activists, these experts could just as easily fight for school choice in inner cities with failing public schools. After all, we know that education is linked to both future earning and health. And wouldn't it make sense to encourage marriage and religious activity, since both are associated with better health?[71] It would, but don't expect to hear as much about these options from the practitioners of PC medicine—they simply do not fit their political agenda.

We must also put into perspective the evidence for a relationship between emotional state and physiology. Numerous studies have documented an association between emotional state, especially anger and hostility, and cardiovascular disease.[72] In an exhaustive book on the topic, *Anger, Hostility and the Heart,* the psychologist Aron W. Siegman classifies two types of anger: withheld anger (also called repressed anger) and expressed anger. Siegman documents scores of studies showing a relationship between both kinds of anger and increased blood pressure, stronger contractility of the heart (sometimes experienced as palpitations) and irregular heartbeats.[73]

S. Leonard Syme of Berkeley's School of Public Health was one of the first to describe the "control of destiny" theory when he examined the landmark Whitehall studies performed by researchers at University College in London.[74] The studies examined workers in the five grades of the British Civil Service, all of whom had access to nationalized health care. While it did not surprise researchers that the civil servants in the lowest grade suffered heart disease at about three times the rate of administrators in the highest, or fifth, stratum, they were puzzled to find that even highly paid professionals in the fourth grade suffered twice as much cardiovascular disease as top-ranking administrators.[75] What appeared to explain this finding was the fact that these professionals had little "control of destiny"—their jobs were fraught with responsibility but they could exercise little authority.

Another term for this phenomenon, discovered independently by the psychologist Martin P. Seligman in his work with animals, is "learned helplessness": a posture of defeat and resignation (often accompanied by physical symptoms) that follows repeated failed attempts by the animal to change its environment. Eventually the animal "learns" to adopt a helpless, passive stance because there is little it can do to influence events. People, too, can become passive when they feel unable to control their lives.

Not all people retreat into passivity, of course, but for those on the threshold of resignation, the indoctrinologists' message of hopelessness in the face of prevailing social conditions is probably the last thing they need to hear. Such defeatism can only encourage the development of learned helplessness and a feeling of lack of "control of destiny." After all, imagine being told that your health is determined by your place on the socioeconomic ladder (which these commentators erroneously assume to be permanent). If you are mired at the bottom, why bother to take care of yourself?

Social production researchers read predictably one-sided interpretations into neutral data. We see this in the use to which evidence of the relationships between health and socioeconomic gradients has been put: as one-sided cautionary tales about the perils of hierarchy. As John W. Lynch and George A. Kaplan of the University of Michigan speculate, "Health may be affected through individual appraisals of relative position in social order. . . . Even those with good incomes might feel 'relatively deprived' compared to the super rich."[76] Richard Wilkinson is more emphatic: "The social consequences of people's differing circumstances in terms of stress, self-esteem and social relations, may be one of the most important influences on health."[77] This assumption leads Wilkinson and others to conclude that a less economically and socially stratified society is a healthier, and hence preferable, society.

But wait a moment. If this so-called relative position theory is true, aren't there alternative lessons to be gleaned? For example, couldn't we just as easily think of the Whitehall study of cardiovascular disease as an object lesson in the importance of free enterprise, accountability and opportunities to be creative on the job? Workers who are responsible for certain tasks would have the latitude to fulfill them, thus minimizing the stress that comes from being stymied when one wants to do a good job. With accountability they could take more pride in what they have accomplished and enjoy enhanced self-esteem. Why overthrow the meritocracy, as Zierler suggests, when reinforcing it—so that people could get results based on their performance—might be a formidable antidote to learned helplessness? The answer by now should be clear: the only acceptable remedies in PC medicine are social actions that would disrupt our prevailing economic and social systems.

In the end, whatever larger social meaning we ascribe to "control of destiny," the consensus among responsible scientists is that chronic, low-grade stress is not good for one's health. The precise mechanism by which "control of destiny" stress might translate into physical damage such as sustained hypertension, heart attack or heart failure is not known, but intriguing data and plausible theories abound.[78] Perhaps there is trauma to the inside of blood vessels from repeated frustration-induced surges in blood pressure. Or perhaps stress disrupts the normal cardiac rhythm, produces a blood vessel spasm or even leads to smoking, which in turn has its own effects on blood pressure.[79] Hormonal, neural and immunologic changes are also probably involved in regulating the cardiovascular system. Although I could find no research on emotional states related to "racism" per se, who could doubt that people who have been discriminated against feel anger (withheld or expressed)? This could conceivably contribute to high blood pressure and other cardiovascular problems.

It is important to remember, however, that the body cannot "tell" where the anger is coming from. Thus, ironically, the anger and stress engendered by being a victim of bias are no different, physiologically speaking, from the anger and stress experienced by the victimizer himself. After all, the classic racist is a seething individual who stews in his hatred until he erupts—that is, he withholds and then expresses rage. This would seem to describe the prototypical "angry white male"—the man who feels that minorities and women are getting ahead at his expense. Is he not a perfect candidate for "low control of destiny"? What's more, this dynamic is by no means limited to black-white interactions. What about the tension and resentment between lighter- and darker-skinned individuals within a minority group?[80]

Granted, it makes a more compelling, and certainly politically correct, story to link the stress in minorities (and subsequent illness) to being a victim of white antipathy, but an evenhanded approach to research on stress and disease cannot be guided by a script. To be sure, researchers should nurture their hunches about the way the world works (it's hard to imagine they could avoid it), but their job is to test these hunches, or hypotheses, by interpreting the data from all angles, not just the ones that mesh with their political philosophy.

Mexican American Women and the Healthy Baby "Paradox"

Many Mexican Americans are found in the lower reaches of the income and education scales, but Mexican American infants are significantly healthier than infants from other low-income groups. The Mexican American infant mortality rate (defined as death before one year of age) was the same as for white babies—almost six deaths per thousand live births—in 1997, according to the National Center for Health Statistics. For Native Americans the rate was slightly under nine deaths per thousand live births, and for black babies almost fourteen.[81]

Health insurance played little role in these differences, since Mexican American women were less likely than other groups to have public or private insurance. Sixty-two percent of them were insured, while 85 percent of white women and 76 percent of both African American and Puerto Rican women were insured. In fact, Mexican American babies were more than twice as likely to be born outside of a hospital compared to babies of all other groups.[82] Among Mexican Americans themselves, we find a difference between the children of recent Mexican immigrants and those of acculturated Mexican Americans. Though the immigrants are poorer and have less education and only tenuous access to health care, their babies weigh more at birth and have a greater chance of surviving their first year than those of U.S.-born mothers of Mexican descent—babies who, in turn, still have lower rates of infant mortality than many other groups in this country.

The health of Mexican American infants, especially the babies of recent immigrants, was so unexpected by researchers that they labeled it the "epidemiological paradox."[83] It seems less paradoxical, however, when we see that the immigrant women have healthier diets and are far less likely to use drugs in pregnancy than their acculturated counterparts.[84] Javier I. Escobar, a psychiatrist at the Robert Wood Johnson Medical School, believes these differences reflect an "acculturation" effect and the erosion of Mexican tradition. "I strongly suspect that the real reason for the advantages that Mexican immigrants have may be . . . a protective or buffering effect of traditional culture," he writes.[85] According to David E. Hayes-Bautista, a professor of medicine at UCLA, Latinos in Los Angeles "have one of the longest life expectancies and lowest disease burdens in spite of their lack of health insurance."[86] Traditionally, the close-knit, extended family networks of Hispanics offer a great deal of support. These bonds break down somewhat once immigrant families are exposed to and absorbed into American culture. Escobar says that lifestyle is also affected—diet becomes less healthy, for instance. Yet some of the beneficial effects of the Mexican heritage linger. Thus, Mexican American babies are better off than those of other groups, but worse off than babies of new immigrants.

It must be noted, however, that familial support, good nutrition and self-care are not always enough to ensure healthy babies. Epidemiologists and pediatricians remain puzzled about the extremely high rate of infant mortality in African American babies: between thirteen and fourteen per thousand live births among African Americans, compared with six to seven per thousand live births in all other groups. The two-to-one mortality pattern persists into the highest reaches of the socioeconomic scale. The Centers for Disease Control and other agencies and research institutions are investigating why the leading causes of infant death, such as birth defects, problems associated with low birthweight and sudden infant death syndrome (SIDS), are more common among black babies.

James W. Collins Jr., a neonatologist at Northwestern University School of Medicine, suggests racism as an underlying cause. "Even if a middle income couple ends up in a comfortable home in an economically stable neighborhood that is not adjacent to a toxic landfill, is the psychosocial cost they pay to overcome racial barriers not of some importance? Indeed, could not this sort of experience have direct adverse health effects?" ask Collins and his colleague R. J. Davis in the article "Bad Outcomes in Black Babies: Race or Racism?"[87] According to Collins and others, the chronic stress induced by racism could elevate hormones that set off premature labor or lower resistance to vaginal infections, also known to be more prevalent among African American mothers.[88]

The theory that disproportionate rates of infant mortality in black babies are attributable to racism-induced stress experienced by the mother has as little empirical foundation as Krieger and Sidney's blood pressure–race discrimination theory. Nonetheless, to the extent that some women, for whatever reason, are at risk for sustained levels of stress during pregnancy, the physiologically buffering effects of good self-care, prenatal checkups, adequate nutrition and abstinence from nicotine, alcohol and drugs become even more important.

Choices and the Health Care System

Even when preventive health services are available, poor and minority individuals tend to make less use of them. For example, when the Breast Examination Center of Harlem began offering free mammograms in 1994, "its doctors were dismayed to discover that the women of Harlem were not banging down their doors," reported the *New York Times*.[89] The experience of Harlem's center is sadly familiar. Poor and minority women often decline offers of a free mammogram.[90] One study found that most of the women who had not obtained one didn't think it was necessary—a reason more commonly given than lack of health insurance or ability to pay.[91] According to a 1993 study reported in *Cancer*, black women are more likely to go to the doctor for treatment of something that is bothering them than for preventive care like screening.[92]

Follow-up rates may differ as well. A number of studies found that white women returned to the doctor for follow-up treatment when a breast cancer abnormality was diagnosed at significantly higher rates than black and Hispanic women.[93] With respect to screening for cervical cancer, another study found that, among women with abnormal Pap smears,

30 to 50 percent never returned to the doctor, and poor and minority women were overrepresented among the no-shows.[94]

This is especially tragic because screening for cervical cancer works. The diagnosis of a pre- or early cancerous state is relatively easy to make, and treatment for early stages of cancer is very effective: 95 percent of women with early cervical cancer are alive five years after diagnosis and treatment. "Part of this has to do with attitude," explains Roshan Bastani, the lead researcher on a UCLA breast cancer study. Bastani found that nearly all white women diagnosed with a breast abnormality followed up, but only 75 percent of black and Hispanic women did, some of them thinking, Bastani says, that "it will go away."[95]

Social networks are important too. According to a study by researchers at the University of California at Berkeley, black women were more likely to undergo a routine mammogram (even after controlling for age, health and insurance status) if they had strong ties to family and community.[96] The researchers concluded that social connections were important in encouraging women not only to seek an initial test but to follow up the results. No doubt these findings extend to women of all races. Some patients put off doctors' appointments because they believe their health is in God's hands. Such fatalism may be especially common among Hispanic patients, explains Clay E. Simpson Jr. of the HHS Office of Minority Health.[97] Native Americans, some unacculturated immigrant groups and populations in the Appalachians may cleave to folk wisdom about health (especially in communities with strong traditions based on such wisdom) and feel intimidated by the health system.

Too many men, especially African Americans, avoid being checked for prostate and colon cancer because of their aversion to the rectal exam and colonoscopy, respectively. The side effects of cancer treatments keep some people from screening (in particular, the high risk of impotence, sometimes irreversible, that accompanies chemotherapy, radiation and surgery for prostate cancer), as do pessimism about surviving cancer and a general lack of information about symptoms, diagnosis and treatment.[98] These factors may explain why black men are more likely to come to their doctors with an advanced stage of prostate cancer even when there is access to care.[99]

Less-educated men and women, whatever their race, may be relatively uninformed about the importance of screening or uneasy with technology. For example, women with under twelve years of education were less likely to have been screened for cervical cancer—or to have even heard of Pap smears—and to have obtained mammograms.[100] In a sample of minority women in Seattle, those who did not get mammograms regularly told researchers that, among other things, they worried that pressure from the machine would cause breast cancer.[101] Says Lorna G. Canlas, a nurse with an East Harlem clinic that cares for a Latino population, "Most clients I encounter need to be persuaded of the validity and utility of modern medical practices."[102]

The phenomenon is not limited to cancer. In Massachusetts and other states, expansion of state-funded prenatal care services did not result in the anticipated increase in use of care or improvement in birth outcomes.[103] Elsewhere, free or low-cost prenatal care was underused.[104] The problem of low regional vaccination rates was discovered to be the result of mothers not bringing their children in for scheduled shots rather than a lack of free vaccination services.[105] Inner-city black patients with HIV/AIDS, according to the New York City Treatment Access Data Network, declined free or low-cost drug therapy; other analyses of patients reporting nonreceipt of drug therapy showed that patients were in fact offered the medications.[106]

Making a Difference at the Front Lines

But there is much that can be done in the areas I've just described, and front-line public health professionals are doing it. Across the country thousands of partnerships between communities (especially churches) and nonprofit health foundations and academic medical centers are under way. Some very practical solutions have emerged—for example, sending personalized reminders for screening in the mail or by phone; televising ads with toll-free numbers for making appointments; and deploying mammography vans.

In 1999 the Boston Public Health Commission launched an aggressive three-point anticancer campaign. First, every Boston household received information on cancer prevention. Second, free and low-cost screening was made available, and municipal employees were allowed to take four (paid) hours off each year for screening. And third, all Bostonians with cancer were provided with transportation to and from chemotherapy, radiation treatments and doctor visits.[107] For the poor, rural population of Birmingham, the University of Alabama helped create a cookbook of heart-healthy meals for church dinners and developed a food stamp program for purchasing fresh produce at local farmers' markets.[108] With less than half of Korean women over fifty being checked for cancer in the past year, the University of California at Berkeley distributed Korean-language educational materials about breast and cervical cancer and held workshops in Korean churches.

Improving health literacy has taken on urgency as well. The American Medical Foundation, the philanthropic arm of the American Medical Association, began efforts to help patients use the drugs they are prescribed after a large study of functional literacy in the United States found that one-third of English-speaking patients could not read or understand directions on prescription bottles, appointment slips and other printed information.[109]

With managed care cutting into doctors' incomes and piling on paperwork, the impulse to provide charity care has diminished considerably over the last decade. From 1993 to 1998 the Robert Wood Johnson Foundation funded Operation Reach Out, which took care of the burdensome paperwork and handled the bureaucracies so that doctors could provide free care with minimal hassle.

One could easily devote a separate volume to the countless educational and health care outreach efforts under way, including public-private partnerships between hospitals and communities. But in the end these services are compensatory, part of the health care safety net.

One problem is that even the best screening services don't help the working poor when a test comes back positive for cancer—they cannot afford the next step: cancer treatment. Dr. Ann S. O'Malley of the Georgetown University Health Center confronts this routinely. Her patients are in the no-win position of having their cancers detected through public screening programs yet depending for treatment on the chance availability of increasingly scarce charity care from physicians and hospitals. To remedy this for women, Congress passed legislation to cover breast and cervical cancer treatment benefits in 2000.

Admittedly, this is not fair to uninsured men who are diagnosed with prostate or colon cancer. "Picking one group over another in addressing problems posed by lack of insurance is a practice that is far from ideal," says O'Malley.[110] Indeed, will we need more piecemeal legislation to ensure cancer treatment for the uninsured? Must we depend on a safety net to catch them and all the others who still fall through the gaps in our private and public insurance systems? Do we need universal health care? These questions won't be resolved anytime soon, but at least they frame an appropriate problem—one with palpable consequences for the health of Americans—for public health experts to tackle.

A Profession Losing Its Moorings?

If the "reallocation of society's resources" and the quest for social justice seem remote from practical public health, policy statements issued by the American Public Health Association show just how far beyond the bounds of clinical relevance the profession has drifted. The association has officially opposed aid to the contras in Nicaragua and war in the Middle East, and it has issued a policy statement for a "nuclear-weapon-free world."[111] On the domestic front, the association has called for congressional campaign finance reform, tried to stymie welfare reform and rejected a proposal for increased state control over Medicaid.[112]

Fernando M. Treviño, a former association president and dean of the public health school at the University of North Texas, assures me that a preoccupation with politics does not reflect the "silent majority of the APHA." Nevertheless, he cautions, "unless the APHA leadership is politically and philosophically in concert with the rank and file, the association runs the risk of becoming irrelevant."[113] That would be a shame, since the rank-and-file members are data-driven professionals who practice traditional public health, like tracking infectious diseases and cancer, protecting us from drug-resistant tuberculosis and bacterial outbreaks after natural disasters and educating communities about ways to reduce the risk of illness. When HIV/AIDS first appeared in the early 1980s, it was these professionals who urged adoption of standard public health procedures while the association as a body remained silent.

The association, like the CDC, the Institute of Medicine, the White House AIDS Office and most gay advocacy groups, struggled with the question of whether concern about the civil rights of gay men should outweigh the opportunity to curtail HIV/AIDS through routine public health maneuvers. The principles at stake were by no means trivial, involving potential discrimination against homosexuals, and especially infected homosexuals, if confidentiality were not tightly preserved. But as Randy Shilts stated in his book *And the Band Played On:* "People died while public health authorities . . . refused to take the tough measures needed to curb the epidemic's spread."[114] As the journalist Chandler Burr noted in his 1997 article "The AIDS Exception," many doctors and public health officials were sympathetic to the gay community's repudiation of the use of tracking and notification practices.[115]

Today there is virtual consensus among public health professionals that we could have limited the AIDS epidemic had some or all of the following steps been taken: (1) routine testing for infection, (2) reporting of positive individuals to the local health department, (3) contact tracing to identify others who may have been exposed (key for babies born to infected mothers since medication can significantly cut the risk of AIDS developing in newborns), and (4) notification of those people. These practices are routinely employed for outbreaks of scores of contagious diseases like tuberculosis, typhoid and syphilis—few of which, unlike HIV/AIDS, are virtually always lethal. Yet as of the spring of 2000 the APHA has been silent on testing newborns for HIV and opposes mandatory testing of pregnant women.[116]

Katherine Marconi, a member of the APHA and director of science and epidemiology at the Health Services Resources Administration, expressed her frustration about the association's pursuit of a larger social agenda. Writing in the association's monthly newspaper, *The Nation's Health,* she asks: "Is there room left in the APHA for health workers who define themselves as conservative or centrist, agree with limitations on abortion or support states' rights? . . . Members come from the whole spectrum of political perspectives. . . . If the 'American' in APHA is forgotten, and the Association's vision centers on politics and not public health, there will be limited room in APHA for its members."[117]

The pursuit of social justice is loosening the public health profession from its scientific and clinical moorings. Certainly, as citizens, public health professionals are free to be active in any political sphere they like, but they must keep their politics from influencing their classroom, their interpretation of research and their health prescriptions. Professionals betray the public's trust when they use their status as health experts to continue the work they began as political activists in the 1960s.

Sometimes it is difficult to know where the boundaries are. I myself may have crossed the line between clinical care and "reform." In the 1994–95 policy debate over whether addiction to drugs and alcohol should be considered a disability by the Social Security Administration, Congress specifically asked whether the individuals concerned should receive income maintenance in the form of cash in the same way that other disabled beneficiaries do. At a congressional hearing I answered no. I had spent years watching cash benefits undermine the work of health professionals. More important, since my patients often spent part or all of their monthly check on cocaine, the cash benefits undermined their expressed desire to quit drugs.

A solution? I suggested that drug treatment compliance be a condition of receiving benefits; that only in-kind, not cash, benefits be distributed, and that time limits be placed on eligibility for "addiction disability" benefits. In other words, the program should be run like a treatment scholarship. Not everyone agreed with my proposal, of course, but it had the advantage of being clinically informed: it was prompted by my experience in the field, and the experiences of others like me, and it was specific. Unlike the indoctrinologists, I was not out to transform the nation's economic and political systems in the name of health; I wanted to push the day-to-day behavior of drug addicts toward the achievable: measurable sobriety and personal productivity.

This is not to deny the existence of social problems in our nation, nor to say that certain social changes couldn't improve the human condition (health included) in the long run. There is no reason, furthermore, why careful research on the relationship between social variables and health should not proceed and quality results be published for the enlightenment of professionals and the lay public alike. But the more passionately public health experts pursue social justice, the less effort, time and money they can devote to promoting health for Americans today. With more than half of all deaths resulting from diseases that are preventable or modifiable, it is indeed reckless to downplay the virtues of self-care.

Worse, putting social justice at the core of the public health enterprise undermines individual accountability. People who practice unsafe sex, stick dirty needles in their veins or fail to take their TB medications daily are too often seen as passive victims of malign social forces. One is accused of "blaming the victim" for expecting them to make safer choices, an expectation that takes on added urgency when third parties are endangered by their behavior. On the contrary, to accept recklessness—or worse, to expect it—is a great disservice to vulnerable people, blinding them to the power they *do* have to enhance their own well-being.

Do I think that public leaders and politicians are going to attempt massive social reforms (for example, by "closing the power gap," "counteracting the free market with social programs" and so on) based on the urging of an activist cohort of public health professors? Of course not. Yet the essence of the indoctrinologists' claim—that being a victim of social forces can make you sick—is not to be dismissed. Victim politics is indeed finding expression in a number of real-world clinical domains.

In the subsequent chapters I use specific examples to show how identity politics has taken precedence over clinical imperatives. I describe how clinical teaching is being politicized, how the importance of personal responsibility for one's health is being undermined and how differences in health outcomes between groups are uncritically accepted as evidence of bias in the health care system. People are often surprised to hear that political correctness is spreading into the clinical arena. But as we will see, not even medicine is immune.

2

Inmates Take Over the Asylum

Around midday on October 5, 1998, forty-six-year-old Margaret Mary Ray set her backpack and purse down by the railroad tracks in a small Colorado town. Then she knelt in front of an onrushing coal train and was instantly killed. Ray, who suffered from schizophrenia, had become infamous for stalking David Letterman, the television personality; she harbored the delusion that she was having a love affair with him. She had once left cookies and an empty whisky bottle in the foyer of the Letterman home in New Canaan, Connecticut.[1]

Ray's history of mental illness had been long and troubled. Since her twenties, she had been in and out of psychiatric hospitals and jails. On antipsychotic medication she did well, but eventually she stopped taking the medicine and quickly deteriorated. Two months before her suicide she was arrested for the last time. At the hearing at which she was freed, the *New York Times* reported, "A judge openly lamented the absence of any legal mechanism to make sure she received medical help."[2]

In fact, such a mechanism does exist. In a form of involuntary treatment called outpatient commitment, a court may order a regime of therapy and medication, and the patient may be rehospitalized if she fails to comply. Because of activism by a small but vocal group of former psychiatric patients, however, supported by civil liberties lawyers, thousands of people like Ray are not receiving the treatment they need to get well or at least to be safe. These activists call themselves "consumer-survivors" (also "psychiatric survivors"). The term "consumer" denotes a user of mental health services, and "survivor" refers to one who has endured psychiatric care. "Survivor" is not used in this term in the same sense as "cancer survivor," someone who has had cancer and survived it, says the psychiatrist and researcher E. Fuller Torrey. "Rather," he points out, "it is being used like 'Holocaust survivor,' an individual who has been unjustly imprisoned and even tortured."[3] Some consumer-survivors have requested that the mental health profession "make an apology to consumers for past abuses of power."[4] As we will see, radical consumer-survivors are the ones who more properly owe apologies to patients for standing in the way of constructive treatments and policies.

Consumer-survivors claim that psychiatrists make them sick. As Coni Kalinowski, a psychiatrist herself, and the consumer-survivor Darby Penney put it, "Ex-patients came to learn that their feelings of isolation, inadequacy, and powerlessness were the result of real practices within the mental health system . . . not . . . products of their illnesses."[5] They point to the deplorable history of the mental health system earlier in the twentieth century, when negligence and even brutality were common in state psychiatric hospitals, but ignore the reforms that have largely eliminated such abuses. The National Association of Consumer-Survivor Mental Health Administrators—a subcommittee of a group called MadNation— wants "an oversight board including consumers and survivors to inspect treatment facilities and mechanisms for grievances" and laws "to limit the powers of psychiatry by making consumers full partners in diagnosing and treatment."[6]

Jackie Parrish, a nurse who formerly served as director of community support programs at the federal Center for Mental Health Services (CMHS), sees this type of partnership as merely a transitional phase. Consumer-survivor involvement in developing state mental health plans is good, Parrish believes, but it "is only an interim step to being totally consumer driven." Optimally, she says, the patients should become "the managers, and administrators—that is what will bring real change."[7]

Parrish envisions peer-run services. Based on relationships of equality between peers, these services are a postmodern alternative to the traditional psychiatrist-patient relationship, which consumer-survivors condemn for perpetuating a "power differential" between the healthy, dominant doctor and the ill, dependent patient.[8] MadNation sponsored an online referendum asking respondents to vote yes or no on the question: "Is the demonization of people diagnosed with mental illness a hate crime?"[9] Cecilia Vergaretti of the Mental Health Association of Oregon extends the battle against "power differentials" beyond the mental health system, which, to her, is merely a microcosm of the larger universe of societal injustice. "This is not about reforming an ailing [mental] health care system," she says, sounding like a professional indoctrinologist. "It's about reforming society."[10]

Do I deny that some mentally ill people have been treated insensitively, even maltreated, by psychiatrists and hospitals? Not for a minute. In fact, I would readily join with consumer-survivors if they worked toward weeding out incompetent clinicians or promoting more vocational rehabilitation, supported housing and so on. But whatever real or perceived injustices have embittered them, we cannot afford to compromise the prospects of severely mentally ill people like Margaret Mary Ray by allowing consumer-survivors to be in charge of others' treatment.

Their Crusade, Your Tax Dollars

Unfortunately, the federal government and state mental health agencies across the country are giving moral and financial support to the consumer-survivor movement. One of the biggest boosters is Bernard Arons, director of CMHS. Under him, CMHS funds the National Empowerment Center, an advocacy organization that is flatly against treatment by psychiatrists. "Our primary physicians must be ourselves," writes Scott Snedecor, program manager of a consumer-operated drop-in center in Portland, Oregon. In his center's newsletter, Snedecor claims that "medication can be worse than psychosis."[11] Pat Deegan, a consumer activist and Snedecor's colleague at the Portland center, is interested in "rehabilitating mental health workers." She produced a project called "Spirit Breaking: How the Helping Professions Hurt."[12] Paolo Del Vecchio, a CMHS consumer affairs specialist, explained to me why he and his colleagues oppose involuntary treatment: it reminds patients of "their own personal Holocaust and leaves them feeling hopeless, believing they will never recover."[13]

Not all people who refer to themselves as "consumer-survivors" are hostile to psychiatry. Take Ken Steele, a fifty-two-year-old New York City man with schizophrenia who was profiled in a front-page story in the *New York Times* and who is writing a book about his life. Steele has no interest in undermining professional care, but he does want to see consumers more actively involved in the system. (Steele himself serves on the boards of several mental health professional organizations.) He sees a psychiatrist and takes an antipsychotic medication called risperidone. When he began the medication in 1995, one year after it came on the market, the unseen voices that he had heard since age fourteen finally ceased. Steele publishes *New York City Voices,* a newspaper about mental health issues, and he counsels and hosts groups for people with schizophrenia to help keep them from lapsing into social isolation.

As a self-identified consumer-survivor, Ken Steele is an asset, not a danger. He is not part of the radical element that denies the reality of mental illness, rejects medication and won't acknowledge the need to step in when individuals are deranged beyond reason. Ken Steele does not want to take over the system. But the radical consumer-survivors, despite their fringe rhetoric and modest head count (they probably total only a few hundred), have infiltrated the mental health system in ways that are truly destructive.

The National Mental Health Consumers' Self-Help Clearinghouse promotes the work of the radical consumer-survivors. It is funded largely by the federal Center for Mental Health Services. In the summer of 1999 the clearinghouse organized the National Summit of Mental Health Consumers and Survivors in Portland, Oregon. Among the major topics were "seclusion and restraint" (the hospital practice of putting violent or out-of-control patients in locked rooms or securing them in bed until they are safe) and outpatient commitment. Both practices were deemed intolerable by the summit leadership.[14]

Consumer-survivors have been spreading the word to other countries as well. In September 1999 a group of fifteen flew to Santiago, Chile, to attend the biannual meeting of the World Federation for Mental Health (an otherwise mainstream conference), courtesy of travel scholarships funded by CMHS. Among the scholarship recipients was David Oaks, director of the National Support Coalition International, based in Eugene, Oregon.

Oaks, a Harvard graduate who suffered a psychotic episode as a young man, is staunchly opposed to psychiatry. He talks about having been a "guinea pig" for doctors prescribing psychiatric drugs ("a hundred times worse than a bad acid trip") and vows to lead a "guinea pigs' rebellion." Oaks insists that mentally ill people can recover through diet, exercise, meditation, writing and peer support.[15] Most dramatically, he claims to have organized what coalition members call an "underground railroad" to help patients cross state lines in order to "escape forced outpatient psychiatric drugging."[16] A month before the Santiago conference, he helped kill several involuntary treatment bills under consideration by the Oregon legislature.[17]

CMHS also publishes the *Consumer Affairs Bulletin,* in which the mental health system (the very system that the center's block grants sustain) is portrayed as heartless and repressive. Here is an excerpt from an item by a consumer-survivor who calls herself Niyyah:

> I would like to share with you what life has been like for myself, my children, and my grandchildren as a consumer-survivor/patient. How race, sex, and disability have hurt us. . . . I believe that racism, stigma, mentalism, poverty, victimization, homelessness, and institutionalization have contributed to a continued intergenerational cycle of needs and dependency. I am a woman who has survived every form of violence known to man, sexual incest . . . ritual abuse, neglect and system abuse. I've also survived what many of us call re-traumatization. This happens when you try to get help and the doctors hurt you again. I've been misdiagnosed, beaten, battered, raped repeatedly, held hostage.[18]

Tax money was also spent to get the consumer-survivor message to Congress and the president via the National Disability Council, an independent federal agency with fifteen presidentially appointed and Senate-confirmed members. The council's recommendations for mental health services, released in early 2000, had the fingerprints of the radical consumer-survivors all over them. This was not surprising since the public hearing at which the council listened to testimony was held on-site at the 1998 annual meeting of the National Association of Rights, Protection and Advocacy, a vigorously antipsychiatry organization.

The title of the council report embodies the ethos of the consumer-survivor movement: "From Privileges to Rights: People Labeled with Psychiatric Disabilities Speak for Themselves."[19] Labeled? In other council documents there is no reference to people labeled with *physical* disabilities. That is because physical disabilities can be seen; it is hard, after all, for any observer to dispute the reality of a wheelchair. But psychiatric diagnoses, consumer-survivors argue, do not exist as fixed and defined entities. They are socially constructed and exist merely in the eyes of the beholders—namely, psychiatrists and other members of the dominant culture.

In a letter to President Clinton, the council tried to portray involuntary treatment as a violation of the Americans with Disabilities Act. "All policies that restrict the rights of people with psychiatric disabilities simply because of their disabilities are inharmonious with basic principles of law and justice, as well as with such landmark civil rights laws as the Americans with Disabilities Act," wrote Marca Bristo, chairperson of the council.[20] The council missed the vital point that psychosis itself, the very justification for involuntary interventions in the first place, can be "inharmonious" with the basic human impulse toward self-preservation. In its zeal to promote alternatives to medical and biochemical approaches (such as so-called peer support), the council denounced electroconvulsive therapy (ECT) and insurance coverage for involuntary hospitalizations.

Alternatives '99: The Guinea Pigs' Rebellion

Since 1985 CMHS has funded an annual consumer-survivors' conference called "Alternatives." At one Alternatives conference a psychologist named Al Siebert presented a talk entitled "Successful Schizophrenia—The Survivor Personality," advertised in the conference program as a discussion of "how schizophrenia is a healthy, valid, desirable condition, not a disorder."[21] According to Siebert: "Schizophrenia has never been proven to be an illness or disease. What is called schizophrenia in young people appears to be a healthy transformational process that should be facilitated instead of treated." How ironic that CMHS is supporting a movement that minimizes the severity of mental illness and discourages the treatments and programs for which CMHS itself, in its role as the government's administrator of public funds for mental health treatment, is paying.

I attended the four-day Alternatives '99 conference in Houston in October of that year. There were seminars on grassroots organizing and on creating openings for consumer-survivors on the boards of managed care organizations and other social services agencies. Consumer-survivors were given ample instruction in how to lobby congresspeople, stop involuntary commitment bills and get more funding from the federal government. Everyone seemed to agree that the state-level success of the consumer-survivor movement had to be replicated at the national level.

There were a number of distractions during the four-day event—poetry readings, clay-molding sessions, group skits. Perhaps appropriately, the nearby Caruso Dinner Theater was putting on a production of *Shear Madness*. I also heard dozens of personal testimonials about the abuses of the "system" and the triumphs of self-help. The "Memorial Wall" was meant to be a palpable reminder of the failure of organized psychiatry. Mounted on three huge poster boards were scores of colored three-by-five cards, each a remembrance of someone who had died. "Dickie Dow, Portland, Oregon. Consumer killed in police custody, Fall 1998," read one. "Rupert: a good friend and next door neighbor—from all of us, Merit Hall, Long Beach." "In Memory of Jacky Jachner: Your star shined brightly, Barbara." It was a sad and touching display, yet I could not help but wonder how many of these people would have still been alive if involuntary treatment laws were more widely in use.

To concede that involuntary treatment is sometimes necessary, however, was beyond the capacity of these consumer-survivors, who already felt so subjugated and powerless. In fact, a major theme of the meeting was that consumer-survivors are the "last minority." "I've always been struck by the similarities between our struggles and those of women, minorities and homosexuals," said Jean Campbell, a consumer-survivor who is on the faculty of the University of Missouri School of Medicine in Columbia. "We are all disempowered, stigmatized, discriminated against, denied our humanity."

There was even a meeting-within-a-meeting called the National People of Color Consumer-Survivor Network, also funded by CMHS. This two-day event was devoted to "learning about the many ways discrimination against consumers exists (e.g., race, ethnicity, sexual orientation, religion, gender, other disabilities, etc.), the 'isms,' and how discrimination and oppression are related to stress."[22]

Sally Zinman of the state-funded California Network of Mental Health Clients attempted to document the experience of being a member of the last minority. In her "study," funded by the state of California, Zinman discovered a "consumer-survivor culture" that was as recognizable as any ethnic culture. After interviewing 135 consumer-survivors in focus group settings, Zinman found that the most frequent self-descriptions were "second-class citizen," "stereotyped" and member of "another civil rights movement." Some spoke of being "celebrated" as mental health clients, and others about the importance of "identify[ing] with their consumer culture."

Zinman works with other diversity trainers (the conventional kind who lecture about African American, Hispanic or Asian American cultures) teaching the personnel in managed care organizations about the consumer culture. A few months before the Alternatives '99 conference, Zinman was one of a group of psychiatric "survivors" invited by Tipper Gore to participate in the White House Conference on Mental Health. Zinman had wanted to engage the vice president's wife in a candid discussion about consumer-survivors and offer her "critiques of a system that often does harm," as she wrote in an op-ed article, but did not get the opportunity.[23]

State-Level Follies

The activists were largely ignored at Mrs. Gore's televised event, but beyond the range of the klieg lights they are wielding influence. By 1997 more than half the states had at least one paid position for a "consumer" in the central office of the state mental health department.[24] So sympathetic to the consumer-survivors was Eileen Elias that during her tenure as Massachusetts commissioner of mental health during the mid-1990s she sent a memo to state hospital staff members instructing them to allow themselves to be put in restraints as an educational exercise.[25] Subsequently, advisers to the National Association for State Mental Health Program Directors suggested that training for physicians, nurses and social workers "might also include such first hand experiences as being admitted to an inpatient facility."[26] Rodney E. Copeland, a psychologist and Vermont's commissioner of mental health, issued a mea culpa to the citizenry in which he said that the mental health profession was guilty of "overemphasis on power, control and paternalism."[27]

State-employed consumer-survivors have access to high-level meetings. Their ability to use the political clout of their departments gives them considerable power over the administration of mental health services. Roughly thirty state mental health authorities have established offices of consumer affairs.[28] These are generally staffed by consumer-survivors whose job, according to CMHS, is to "support consumer empowerment and self-help in their particular states."[29] Federal block grants to states require the establishment of a mental health planning council in each state to monitor the allocation and adequacy of mental health services. At least half of the council staff members must be "adults with serious mental illness who are receiving (or have received) mental services" or family members of such people.[30] At the federal level, CMHS created the Consumer/Survivor Subcommittee to assist its own National Advisory Council. "The creation of this subcommittee is a landmark occasion," said CMHS Director Bernard Arons. "[It] continues our efforts to promote consumer/survivor participation at every level of the mental health system."[31]

Ideologues committed to the consumer-survivor ethos are often put in charge of state offices of patient affairs. Darby Penney, the director of recipient affairs of the New York State Office of Mental Health and a member of MadNation's steering committee, is one. In 1992 she was appointed by the commissioner of mental health, Richard C. Surles, to advise him on the perspectives of consumer-survivors in policymaking. By numerous reports, she has consistently used her position to thwart compulsory treatment.

This was the experience of Paul F. Stavis, a lawyer who served as chief counsel of the New York State Commission on the Quality of Care for the Mentally Disabled. In 1995 Stavis was asked by Governor George Pataki to head an investigation of a high-profile killing by Ruben Harris, a forty-two-year-old man with a long history of schizophrenia and violence. He had run away from the Manhattan Psychiatric Center, stopped his medication and started using drugs. Ten days later he pushed Soon Sin, a Korean grandmother, into the path of a subway train.

"We did our review and advised the Office of Mental Health to compel high-risk patients to stay on the treatment regimens," Stavis told me. The recommendation was straightforward: simply revive the law on "conditional release," which had been on the books since 1919. This would allow a director of a psychiatric facility to release a psychotic patient, once successfully treated, on the condition that he complied with medication and other necessary treatment. The conditions could include abstaining from illicit drugs and alcohol as well. If the patient violated the agreement, he would be returned to the facility. "Penney fought us all the way," Stavis recalls, "and in the end she prevailed upon the commissioner to disregard our proposal."[32]

In 1996 I tried to communicate with Penney for an article I was writing. In response to my e-mail, in which I identified myself as a psychiatrist, she wrote that she could see no point in continuing the exchange because, as a psychiatrist, I couldn't possibly understand the consumer perspective. I tried again while working on this book, but she refused to communicate with me. Shutting down conversation is something Penney does with regularity, a number of people told me—all of whom, save Stavis, were unwilling to be identified. She has been known to burst into tears during meetings with state administrators; at one meeting she became so agitated over the use of the word *asylum*—to denote refuge and protection for the mentally ill—that the meeting was derailed and nothing got accomplished.

Penney is often characterized as intolerant of all consumers except those who share, in the words of one critic, her "antipsychiatrist, anti-medication and anti-treatment agenda." She believes that mental illness is a psychological disturbance brought on by abuse—first propagated by one's family, then society, and ultimately the system intended to treat it. It would seem that the best treatment, in her view, is rights advocacy. "Since Penney doesn't believe in treatment," one New York City psychiatrist told me, "how can she be in a position to promote quality in treatment services?" Other colleagues have wondered whether politicians and administrators endorse Penney's rhetoric as an excuse to avoid spending money on the costly needs of the mentally ill—an allegation fit for a tenacious investigative journalist.

It is important to understand that radical consumer-survivors have financial interests to protect as well. Through CMHS, they can apply for funds to develop "peer-run programs." Applicants can also receive money to establish "national technical assistance centers" and "state network grants," the goals of which, according to "Guidance for Applicants," are to foster the "leadership skills of consumer organizations . . . [and] improve communication and cooperation among stakeholders and advocates in the mental health system."[33] According to the National Association of State Mental Health Program Directors, New York State awarded $5 million to consumer-run organizations in 1995, New Jersey $1.6 million and Tennessee $1.2 million.[34]

I should affirm my conviction here that individuals who have in the past been very ill with psychotic or severe mood disorders can do much that is positive. Ken Steele, for example, lectures to patient groups, family members and the public on the importance of medication compliance. Others occupy advisory spots with local mental health agencies; there is a group called Schizophrenics Anonymous. The difference between these individuals and members of the radical consumer-survivor movement is that they want to make the current system function better, not tear it down. Toward that end, they use public funds constructively—for example, to sponsor drop-in centers, clubhouses, employment services and self-help groups, which can provide desperately needed opportunities for socialization and morale-building.

The problem is that consumer-run organizations vary greatly in quality. "When government agencies first started to involve former patients in the early eighties in order to help in planning community services, I thought it was a good idea," Fuller Torrey tells me. "The tragedy is that the effort got hijacked by bureaucrats who were antipsychiatry and naturally gave funding to activist patients."[35] Mentally ill individuals take a considerable risk if they mistakenly join one of the organizations that puts victim politics before their own clinical best interests, like the ones that actively discourage patients from cooperating with the conventional mental health system and from taking medication.

It is certainly true that some of the older antipsychotic medications like Thorazine, Mellaril and Haldol were once given in doses considered too high by today's standards. Psychiatrists used to increase doses abruptly; now it is done more gradually. The side effects suffered by many patients, such as oversedation, "cotton-headedness," muscle stiffness and tardive dyskinesia—uncontrollable movements of the mouth and other parts of the body—made them understandably leery of those medications. Now dosing schedules are more refined, and the new antipsychotics produce fewer disabling side effects. But many consumer-survivors who had bad experiences with medication in the 1970s and 1980s are fighting an image of pharmacotherapy that no longer applies. They don't realize—or don't want to realize—how much things have changed.

Not Really All That Sick

One might reasonably ask: Could someone like Margaret Mary Ray, David Letterman's stalker, hold a responsible position in a government agency? Of course not. And therein lies one of the problems with the radical consumer-survivor movement. Its leaders are relatively well functioning, as mental patients go. I could find no systematic survey of the diagnoses or current symptom profile of the movement's most active members, but it is safe to say that their activities require the energy, focus and coherence that elude people who are hallucinating, incoherent, clinically paranoid or unable to concentrate.

The radical consumer-survivors spend much of their time speaking to audiences, mobilizing activists, applying for grant money, organizing and attending conferences, lobbying politicians and advising state and federal agencies involved with treatment and disability rights. All the while, many are receiving disability payments because they consider themselves too ill to hold a job. Yet they manage to marshal their resources in the effort to preserve the "right" of psychotic people to refuse medication, to ensure that hospitals abandon the use of restraints and to overturn outpatient commitment laws. In doing so, they work against the best interests of those who are most seriously ill—those too psychotic to competently refuse medication, too aggressive or confused to be safe without restraint and too unreliable to take the medications that keep them from lapsing back into psychosis.

Bernard Zuber, for one, is appalled by the rhetoric of activists who presume to speak for him. In 1952, when he was nineteen and living in Paris, he tried suicide by hurling himself backward into the path of a taxi. He spent eight years, from 1982 to 1989, in and out of psychiatric hospitals and jails, setting small fires, homeless and filthy on the street. ("I looked like Anthony Hopkins in the movie *Instinct*.")[36]

Then Zuber was admitted to the West Los Angeles Veterans' Hospital. He had cellulitis (infection of the skin) and was malnourished; he stayed mute and curled in a fetal position, refusing to eat. He denied wanting to kill himself because, as he told psychiatrists, "I'm already dead," convinced he had been killed years before under the wheels of that Parisian taxi. Clearly he was in no position to give informed consent for treatment and would have died had his psychiatrists not petitioned the court to authorize surgery for an intestinal blockage that developed during the hospitalization. It was not until 1990 that the doctors diagnosed bipolar disorder; before then his diagnosis had been depression.

Today Zuber works as a clerk for a state agency. As an active member of the California National Alliance for the Mentally Ill (NAMI), he also supports involuntary treatment—he credits it with saving his life. He is dismayed by the efforts of a man named Ron Schraiber, who is the director of the Office of Consumer Affairs of the Los Angeles County Department of Mental Health. Zuber says that Schraiber is supposed to be advising the state's mental health director about helping people like him but instead is fighting against involuntary care. "Schraiber and the other consumer-survivors portray a medical issue as a civil rights issue," Zuber told me. "Some even say they don't believe in the 'medical model' of mental illness. So what was happening to me? There wasn't something wrong with my brain? I just decided to live a certain way? Oh, please."

Moe Armstrong, a fifty-four-year-old resident of Cambridge, Massachusetts, with schizophrenia, agrees with Zuber on the issue of compulsory care. Armstrong spent roughly a dozen years in mental facilities. Many "professional consumers," as he calls them, really "don't have enough contact with sick people, and so they are not a true voice for us."[37] Some people simply need to live in state hospitals, he insists, or should be highly supervised in programs like outpatient commitment.

Consumer-survivors, on the other hand, maintain that anyone can live independently with proper community supports that are individualized to the patient, including modified vehicles and other special equipment, no matter what the cost. Robert E. Nikkel, a social worker, and his colleagues describe the consumer-survivor mind-set in an article in *Psychiatric Services:* "Living in the community is viewed as a civil right and a necessary antidote to the victimization, subtle and not-so-subtle, that has accompanied the status of mental patient in most Western industrialized cultures."[38]

As the National Empowerment Center's director, Daniel B. Fisher, a physician and former psychiatric patient, proclaims: "We are not cases, and we do not want to be managed. Instead we seek to work with personal care attendants like people with other disabilities."[39] The state of Massachusetts shows how far accommodation can go: it actually bought a patient a house and supplied him with attendants twenty-four hours a day.[40] He needed round-the-clock monitoring because one manifestation of his mental condition was habitual fire-setting. The psychiatrist Jeffrey L. Geller, then medical director of the county adjacent to the one in which this patient resided, calculated that the arrangement cost $150,000 a year—more than three times the cost of supervising and caring for this individual in the state hospital.

Independent living proved deadly for Shirley Mattos of Modesto, California. In 1993 the thirty-eight-year-old Mattos was set up in a board-and-care home where she was to be under constant observation by case workers. A few months earlier, according to an account in the *Los Angeles Times*, Mattos was admitted to Napa State Hospital because she had an odd habit of swallowing objects such as pens and pencils when she became angry or frustrated.[41] Having undergone more than fifty operations to remove these objects, she still wanted to live independently. About a year after Mattos and her lawyer secured her discharge from Napa State (over the objections of her psychiatrists), she swallowed a pencil and died soon after having surgery to remove it. "That year," said Dan Pone, Mattos's lawyer, "was probably one of the best, if not the best year, of her life. She was able to live out her dream."

Even for patients who do not require protection from themselves, independent living is not always the best approach. "It can be devastatingly lonely and isolated," Armstrong says. "Some people actually prefer a sanctuary—not all, but some." He thinks the mental health system needs "more humanity," but he doesn't want it dismantled. "I'll need medication and supervision for the rest of my life; I freely admit it. I wish others would."

The state agencies and politicians are making a grave error in assuming that those who claim to represent consumers are actually representative of them, explains D. J. Jaffe, a founder of the Treatment Advocacy Center, which advocates the benefits of involuntary treatment for the severely mentally ill. "The people I most worry about are the ones who are too psychotic to even know they are ill," Jaffe says.[42]

That describes roughly half of all individuals with schizophrenia. But the consumer-survivors would let people like Larry Hogue run free. Dubbed the "Wild Man of Ninety-sixth Street," Hogue terrorized the Upper West Side of Manhattan in the early 1990s by screaming at people, lunging out at them from between parked cars and destroying property. Homeless and mentally ill, he became violent when he used crack cocaine, but local judges released him to the streets as soon as he was not overtly dangerous. Upon release he would stop his medication, use cocaine and end up back in jail or in the psychiatric emergency room in a cycle that went on for years.

Or consider the case of Joyce Brown, who in 1987 became a test case for civil liberties. Homeless and wildly psychotic, screaming obscenities and smeared with her own excrement, Brown (who called herself Billie Boggs) was taken against her will to New York's Bellevue hospital. In the legal battle over whether Brown, forty years old at the time, could be released, the presiding judge, Robert Lippman, sided with Brown, who called herself a political prisoner and was represented by the New York Civil Liberties Union (NYCLU). Society, not Brown, was sick, Judge Lippman insisted, declaring that "the blame and shame must attach to us."[43] After her discharge, the NYCLU employed her for a while as a receptionist. It also helped arrange a speaking engagement for her at Harvard Law School; the title of her talk was "The Homeless Crisis: A Street View."

Soon, however, Brown was back living over the steam grate she called home. For a while in the early 1990s her family had no idea where she was, but acquaintances told the *New York Times* that she lived in a group home.[44] She was back at Bellevue at least once, but as of the spring of 2000 she was not in an institution, according to Norman Siegel of the NYCLU.[45] As he had promised Joyce Brown, he would not give out details about whether she was working or living in a group home.[46] Some have wondered whether she suffered from her brush with fame. "All the exposure, going to Harvard and all, in the end was very detrimental in terms of coming to terms with who she really is," says Joan Olson, director of an agency that once provided housing for Brown. Robert Gould, Brown's former psychiatrist, agrees. "In retrospect, it was too much."[47]

A Brief History of Consumerism

The radical consumer-survivor movement grew out of the 1960s liberationist ethos, which saw mental patients as a class of social dissident and psychiatry as an agent of social control. In the words of the Marxist social critic Herbert Marcuse, psychiatry was seen as "one of the most effective engines of suppression." Explanations for the origins of psychosis abounded. Some implicated psychiatry itself. According to Erving Goffman, author of the influential *Asylums* (1961), the mental hospital itself imposed "abasements, degradation, humiliation and profanations of the self," reinforcing the psychopathology it was meant to cure. R. D. Laing, a

Scottish psychiatrist, thought of psychosis as a rational adaptation to an insane world. In the popular culture, films like *King of Hearts* (1966) and books like Ken Kesey's *One Flew over the Cuckoo's Nest* (1962) sentimentalized the insane as embodying truth, spontaneity and innocence, their souls crushed by stone-hearted authoritarians. "Every psychotic is a potential sage or healer," wrote the physician Andrew Weil, later famous as an alternative medicine guru, in his 1972 book *The Natural Mind.*

By 1974 the number of patients in psychiatric hospitals had been more than halved, from slightly more than five hundred thousand in the mid-1950s. Once released, many of these ex-patients gravitated to one another. "In daily life they were shunned and stigmatized," write Rael Jean Isaac and Virginia Armat in *Madness in the Streets.* They found solace in "an ideology that cast them as romantic figures combating oppression, individuals whose perceptions of the world had equal if not greater validity than those of 'sane' society."[48]

The Insane Liberation Front was founded in 1970 in Portland, Oregon. In 1971 the Mental Patients Liberation Project and the Mental Patients Liberation Front appeared in New York and Boston, respectively. The next year former patients in San Francisco organized the Network Against Psychiatric Assault and the Madness News Network. The first Conference on Human Rights and Psychiatric Oppression was held in Detroit in 1973. Today the most vocal antipsychiatry consumer-survivor groups are the National Empowerment Center near Boston, the National Association for Rights Protection and Advocacy in Rapid City, South Dakota, and the Support Coalition in Eugene, Oregon.

Working with civil liberties lawyers and patients' rights groups like the Mental Health Law Project (which changed its name to the Bazelon Center for Mental Health Law in 1993), activists have lobbied to scale back commitment laws and block involuntary treatment laws from being passed or implemented. They have championed the right of severely ill patients to refuse treatment (representing the expressed wishes of their client-patients even when they are delusional) and campaigned against electroconvulsive therapy.[49] They have succeeded in getting lawmakers in a number of states, including California, Massachusetts, Tennessee and

Texas, to collaborate in writing and, in some cases, passing legislation restricting the availability of ECT.[50]

ECT, or shock therapy, has a bad public image, crystallized in many minds by the horrific scene in the 1975 film version of *One Flew over the Cuckoo's Nest*. In fact, ECT is one of the most effective treatments available for severe depression. Yet major public hospitals, including Bellevue, Coney Island, Kings County and Woodhull Hospitals in New York City, have stopped performing ECT because of pressure from consumer groups.[51] When the first-ever surgeon general's report on mental health, issued in 1999, gave a clean bill of health to ECT, the consumer-survivor community was livid, the *New York Times* reported.[52] "Your lies threaten to re-traumatize these survivors," fumed David Oaks in a letter to the surgeon general.[53]

Consumer-survivor ideology has found expression in the Protection and Advocacy for the Mentally Ill programs (P&A) created by Congress in 1986. Like so many other consumer-survivor–friendly enterprises, it is funded by CMHS. The fifty protection and advocacy programs, one for each state, were created to investigate allegations of abuse and neglect of mental patients in hospitals and group homes. Federal regulations required that protection and advocacy programs establish a mental health advisory council and that 60 percent of the council membership be current or former psychiatric patients or their family members—a good many of whom, no doubt, offer useful suggestions.

Indeed, many protection and advocacy programs have scored important victories, uncovering serious cases of mistreatment and enacting some valuable reforms. The New York State program, for example, was responsible for making Clozaril, a highly effective but expensive antipsychotic drug, available to patients on Medicaid. But in some other states the protection and advocacy programs have collaborated with civil liberties lawyers to obstruct patients' access to care. In late 1999, for example, Vermont's P&A managed to overturn a law making it easier to medicate psychotic individuals.[54] In New Jersey, P&A lawyers abandoned a short-lived hospital monitoring program and instead returned to advising patients of their legal right to demand release and refuse medication.[55]

A tragic example of P&A intrusion occurred in Texas in 1987. Despite a mother's warning to the P&A agency that her hospitalized (and suicidal) daughter wanted to leave the San Antonio state hospital, a P&A lawyer went to the daughter, ascertained her desire to leave and then represented her. After her discharge was secured, the daughter killed herself. This story was reported to the authors of *Madness in the Streets* by Carmen Johnson, one of the few members of the Texas P&A advisory board who was not a recovering mentally ill person. What floored Johnson even more than the girl's release and subsequent suicide was the board's reaction: they reported it as a "successfully closed case."[56]

The American Psychiatric Association has also objected to the priorities of many P&A lawyers. "We are deeply concerned," the association wrote in 1995 in a letter to Bernard Arons of CMHS, "that the critical element of protecting patients has been seriously under-emphasized."[57] Little has changed, however. The P&A's response to outpatient commitment has exemplified their practice of sacrificing protection for advocacy. An item in the newsletter of the National Association of Protection and Advocacy Systems, *Protection and Advocacy Systems News,* rhetorically asks whether outpatient commitment is "Prescription or Persecution?" and answers, implicitly, that it is the latter.[58]

When P&A agencies have been unable to derail commitment policies outright, they have had no choice but to adopt the role of watchdog, making sure the policies are fairly and efficiently applied. Ironically, it is just this kind of oversight that P&A agencies should have embraced as their job in the first place and that Congress intended as their mission all along. Unfortunately, time and money have been wasted on their initial efforts to defeat outpatient commitment.

Politicians are exceedingly vulnerable to pressure from consumer-survivor groups. Although they make strange bedfellows indeed, budget-conscious politicians who want to save money are sympathetic to advocates who want to dismantle the expensive state institutions. Legislators get understandably nervous when told that their constituents' rights are being trampled, but they rarely know enough about the management of severe mental illness to evaluate the consumer-survivors' histrionic claims of having been abused through involuntary treatment policies. Such claims make them quick to grant concessions. In instances where actual abuse or neglect has been uncovered, politicians are again quick to take the advice of vocal consumer-survivor groups, not realizing that their recommendations will only create more problems.

The Commonsense Family Movement

One of the voices against the antipsychiatry extremism of consumer-survivors is the so-called family movement, led by the National Alliance for the Mentally Ill. Begun in 1978 by parents seeking services for their severely mentally ill children, NAMI and the consumer-survivors have clashed bitterly over the virtues of involuntary treatment. The alliance lobbies for treatment services and research into diseases like schizophrenia and bipolar illness and is vocal about tightening involuntary treatment laws. It has 195,000 members, 70 percent of whom have adult children suffering from schizophrenia or bipolar illness.[59]

Consumer-survivors paint NAMI as a bunch of parents seeking to control their children, in part, to alleviate their own guilt at having raised a child who developed a mental illness. Sylvia Caras, a disability rights advocate and former psychiatric patient in Santa Cruz, California, says that families find "exoneration" when medications are prescribed for their children. Pharmacology then becomes the parents' way to "medicate social disarray." Caras has felt "their shunning since I started publicly to reformulate what I thought about my own experiences with the mental health system." She accuses families who commit relatives to treatment of trying to silence them. Because these families acknowledge the occasional need for restraints, sedation or seclusion, Caras accuses them of endorsing practices that have a "chilling effect on civil rights." Today's mental health approaches, she declares, "will be remembered along with the Salem witchcraft trials as a dishonorable scape-goating of transformative experiences."[60]

Consumer-survivors also lobby strenuously against extending insurance coverage, including Medicare and Medicaid, to hospitals that care for involuntarily committed patients. The Anti-Psychiatry Coalition, a midwestern volunteer group of "people who feel we have been harmed by psychiatry," goes a step further. Oddly enough, the group lobbied hard in Massachusetts to defeat a bill that would have required that psychiatric services be covered on the same basis as other medical and surgical care. As the coalition proclaimed:

> Mental health parity [coverage] will encourage more human rights violations: unnecessary psychiatric incarceration ("hospitalization"), harmful psychiatric drugs unnecessarily imposed on people against their will, more brain-damaged people by psychiatry's drugs and electroshock . . . more people with unjustified psychiatric stigma for the remainder of their lifetimes. Contrary to popular belief, psychiatry is not health care. It is a form of social control.[61]

Radical consumer-survivors can be counted on to reject virtually any good idea that NAMI favors. Mental health courts are one such innovation. The first one was started in Broward County, Florida, in 1997. The courts are a diversionary program for mentally ill nonviolent offenders; instead of going to jail, they are "sentenced" to treatment, and the judge keeps a close eye on the patient-offender to make sure he complies.[62]

With about 10 to 15 percent of jail inmates nationwide known to be mentally ill individuals who were arrested for disruptive behaviors that could have been controlled with medication or supervision, these courts could make a real impact. Patient-offenders could be ushered into supervised treatment and kept out of jail (where they are often brutalized by other inmates). Meanwhile, jail crowding would be relieved. And the crowding can be extreme. "The nation's largest mental institution," is how the *New York Times* referred to the Los Angeles County jail.[63] On any given day in the spring of 2000, it held more than two thousand inmates who suffered from severe mental illness. The largest mental institution in California, Patton State Hospital in San Bernardino County, has around twelve hundred patients.[64]

Mental health courts are gaining popularity. There are plans in Congress to offer grants through the U.S. Attorney General's Office to set up and evaluate twenty-five of the courts between 2000 and 2005. King County in Washington State unveiled its mental health court in the winter of 1999, and the NAMI of Multnomah County, Oregon, has proposed establishing one. The Oregon proposal immediately sparked panic in the state's consumer-survivor community. What's next, asked Pat Risser, a consumer-survivor, "'African-American' courts, or maybe 'gay and lesbian' courts?"[65] Judi Chamberlin of the National Empowerment Center nominated "apartheid courts."[66] These fill-in-the-victim suggestions reflect the consumer-survivors' collective self-image as "the last minority."[67]

The Consumer-Survivor Code of Silence

To be sure, not all psychiatric patients oppose involuntary treatment, reject psychiatric medication or regard mental illness as a transformative experience. "You get excommunicated from the consumer-survivor movement if you speak against the status quo," says Eve, a former psychiatric patient who works with a visiting nurse service in New York City.[68] Most of her patients suffer from schizophrenia or manic-depressive illness. Thirty-eight, married and the mother of a seven-year-old daughter, Eve spent much of her late adolescence institutionalized. After her daughter was born, her postpartum depression was treated with ECT. Several years later she suffered another bout of depression and agreed to have ECT again. Now she takes an antidepressant and a mood stabilizer and is doing well. Like Ken Steele, she calls herself a consumer-survivor, but unlike Steele, Eve feels that she has to go along with the party line. She refused to let me use her real name.

Eve was once active with the radical consumer-survivor movement but has pulled back because, she says, it is "too closed-minded." Still, she is reluctant to disagree openly lest she be frozen out altogether. She departs from the consumer-survivor party line in two ways. She favors involuntary commitment (about half of her patients are under court order to receive treatment and take medications), and she sees value in ECT. Eve

tells of a tenant of a housing program who stopped his antipsychotic medication, began hallucinating and went back to using crack cocaine. Psychotic and aggressive, he got into a fight and broke his arm—a stroke of
luck since it landed him in the hospital. Otherwise, Eve says, the housing
director would have "just let him deteriorate, because that was what her
politics said she should do." Eve didn't protest—she knew it wasn't right
to let the man remain so sick, but she also didn't want to get fired for being
a troublemaker.

It is at this level of day-to-day management that ideology overrides
clinical judgment, with frightening consequences. Many clinicians
report similar stories: patients stop taking their medication and then become too psychotic to remain in supervised housing. The "compassionate" response of the consumer-friendly management has been to *evict*
these patients rather than obtain court orders for treatment. Consumer-
survivor advocacy groups like the Bazelon Center for Mental Health Law
insist that treatment not be required as a condition of residence, and
they are quite adept at creating legal and political obstacles for facilities
that disagree.[69]

In their essay "Housing as a Tool of Coercion," Henry Korman and
his colleagues at Cambridge and Somerville Legal Services in Massachusetts denounce residence contracts that require treatment. While they
properly stress that treatment plans must be flexible enough to accommodate changes in a person's clinical status, they fail to realize that individuals sometime require involuntary treatment to remain stable. "The
only real means of ending compelled acquiescence to treatment in [resi-
dential facilities] is to separate housing from receipt of services," they
write. "Principles of equal treatment . . . forbid intrusion into the zone of
privacy defined by the home."[70]

Thus, Korman effectively undercuts the value of specialized housing
for the mentally ill. His impractical, rights-based solution would take us
back to the days when the mental health system was hopelessly fractured
(more so than it is today) and thousands of sick people dropped through
the cracks and onto the streets. Furthermore, a lax housing scheme spells
disaster for public relations. For example, when the consumer-run Col-

laborative Support Programs Inc. tried to establish a residence in a Clifton, New Jersey, neighborhood in 1998, the townspeople refused to allow it.[71] They knew that program housing did not have a treatment requirement, and they had visions of unmedicated patients wandering the neighborhood or, worse, becoming aggressive—a scenario that might well have come to pass had Korman's vision been realized.

Denying the Reality of Mental Illness

The vast majority of severely mentally ill people can lead safe and comfortable lives in the community as long as they continue to take medication to control such psychotic symptoms as hallucinations and delusional thinking. Without medication, however, they risk the fate of Margaret Mary Ray. That's why outpatient commitment was developed. Such intervention can also interrupt the downward spiral into violence. True, only a small percentage of psychotic individuals ever inflict serious bodily harm—and when they do, it is mostly upon other family members—but the assaults and killings that do occur are tragedies that often could have been avoided.

The potential for violence is a reality of some types of mental illness. In 1998, however, a MacArthur Foundation study found no difference in commission of violent acts between a sample of mentally ill people and the general population. This was a predictable finding, since the study largely excluded subjects with the greatest potential for aggression, but it was touted as a refutation of the "myth" that mentally ill people pose a greater threat than the rest of us. "It's time we kill our cultural fantasy of deranged psychotic killers on the loose," said the president of the National Mental Health Association following the study's publication in the *Archives of General Psychiatry*.[72]

But the well-documented fact is that psychotic individuals not taking medication are indeed more prone to violence. Thirty years of data show this. A study of three hundred patients discharged from California's Napa Valley State Hospital between 1972 and 1975 showed that their arrest rate for violent crimes was ten times higher than that of the general population.[73] In Finland the risk of committing homicide was seven to ten times greater among individuals with schizophrenia than it was among the general population.[74] According to the Department of Justice, approximately one-quarter of all offspring who kill their parents have a history of serious mental illness.[75] As Professor John Monahan of the University of Virginia School of Law summed it up:

> The data that have recently become available, fairly read, suggest the one conclusion I did not want to reach: Whether the measure is the prevalence of violence among the disordered or the prevalence of disorder among the violent, whether the sample is people who are selected for treatment as inmates or patients in institutions or people randomly chosen from the open community, and no matter how many social and demographic factors are statistically taken into account, there appears to be a relationship between mental disorder and violent behavior.[76]

After years of denying the association between untreated mental illness and aggression, the National Alliance for the Mentally Ill has come full circle. Carla Jacobs, an alliance board member from California, became an activist for involuntary commitment after her mother-in-law was fatally stabbed and shot by a mentally ill relative. "We used to think it was stigmatizing to acknowledge violence," Jacobs tells me. "Now we recognize that violence by the minority tars the majority and makes communities less likely to welcome the community-based housing that can facilitate treatment and reduce violence." Too many of our relatives are hurting others and winding up in jail, she laments. "The first step to helping the mentally lies in admitting there is a problem."[77]

The connection between certain types of severe mental illness and violence would seem to be a matter of common sense. But before the 1960s, when deinstitutionalization began in earnest, most of the severest cases were kept out of sight and the public forgot how volatile psychotic people can be. In the 1970s patients' rights activists tried to reduce the stigma of mental illness and thus downplayed the risk of violence. As they became better organized and more influential, the old commonsense view became increasingly controversial.

Am I saying that we need to reinstitutionalize on a grand scale? Not at all. But more states do need to enact laws that protect the person who is not yet helpless or dangerous but, as his family, doctors or local police know from past experience, is likely to deteriorate unless treated. A number of states allow authorities to hospitalize such people against their will, but judges are notoriously reluctant to do so. States should uniformly require judges to consider past violence when deciding about commitment. With most P&As lobbying to maintain the status quo, Congress should change the P&A charter so that these programs no longer perform "A" (advocacy) but focus exclusively on "P" (protection).

Obviously, treatment and specialized social services are of profound importance. There are still gaping holes in the treatment network in most states, and we desperately need more community-based housing and case worker programs. Insurance companies and the public hospital system, for example, routinely refuse to let patients stay in the hospital long enough to recover from a crisis. Even fixing such holes in the system, however, wouldn't eliminate the need for involuntary treatment policies. Granted, the better the mental health system, the less the need for coercion, but that need will never go away entirely. Many people who are actively psychotic have little awareness of their condition. Others know they need help but are too paranoid to seek it out. Even when medicated some remain unaware of their illness (though they feel much calmer and are less symptomatic). These people are not avoiding treatment because of the embarrassment of the "stigma" of schizophrenia, as is the popular belief among even mainstream mental health advocacy groups like the National Mental Health Association. The truth is that they don't even know they are ill.

In 1989 Jonathan Stanley found himself standing naked on a milk crate in the middle of a Manhattan delicatessen. As he tells it: "Secret agents had been chasing me through the streets of New York for three straight days and nights. They had finally cornered me. Only the plastic milk crate insulated me from the deadly radiation aimed at the deli from the satellite dish across the street." Stanley was diagnosed with bipolar illness. With treatment, he was able to go to law school and graduate. "Without treatment, my world would be one of psychosis and delusion," he says. "I would most likely be homeless, in jail or dead."[78]

Frederick Frese, diagnosed with schizophrenia, tells this story:

> I was first diagnosed with paranoid schizophrenia at the age of twenty-five and experienced a series of some ten inpatient stays during the following decade. All but one admission was voluntary. I personally feel that I greatly benefited from being forced to accept treatment during periods in which I was incapable of under-standing that I needed it. In fact, sometimes I wonder what would have become of me had someone not given me the treatment I so desperately needed but was so opposed to accepting.[79]

Frese's recovery, incidentally, was so spectacular that he went on to earn a doctorate in psychology and now works in a state hospital.

Not everyone who is taken to the hospital unwillingly, however, is later thankful. I remember Karen, a young woman with schizophrenia who struggled with the policeman who brought her into our emergency room. She could have easily been arrested for disturbing the peace since she had been throwing garbage at passersby and screaming at the top of her lungs. I wanted to admit her to the hospital, but Karen insisted on going back to the New Haven streets, though the temperature was four degrees and she had no money. To make matters worse, she thought that Agent Mulder of the TV show *The X-Files* was protecting her from being vaporized. So I committed her to the hospital. A week later she was still angry at me for making her stay in the hospital, but at least she had started taking her medication again and agreed to enter a group home.

As long as there is severe mental illness, there will always be people like Karen. But data suggest that most patients who are coerced into the hospital will acknowledge that they needed the care. One recent study in the *American Journal of Psychiatry* interviewed patients two days after admission and then again several weeks later.[80] At two days almost half of all patients admitted involuntarily said that they had needed to be admitted. Only 5 percent had changed their minds when interviewed again several weeks later. Of the patients who initially felt that they did not need to be admitted (about 52 percent), roughly half had changed their minds a few weeks after admission, saying that the decision to hospitalize them against their will was justified. Thus, over three-quarters of the study sample ultimately felt that their treatment had been warranted—though few expressed gratitude as effusively as Stanley and Frese, the researchers pointed out.

The Bellevue Experience

Most states permit outpatient commitment, although it is employed only sporadically. Paul S. Applebaum of the University of Massachusetts School of Medicine in Worcester warned in 1986 that outpatient commitment could have demonstrated value only if the civil liberties lawyers cooperated by realistically assessing the needs of their clients.[81] After longtime resistance to the passage of outpatient commitment legislation, the New York Civil Liberties Union, the Mental Hygiene Legal Service (a nonprofit advocacy group) and the New York State Bar Association's Committee on Mental and Physical Disability finally agreed to a law establishing a limited pilot program in 1994.

In 1995 New York initiated a pilot project at Manhattan's Bellevue Hospital to see whether court-ordered treatment and intensive outpatient services reduced hospital stays for severely mentally ill people with a history of disastrous consequences when they stopped their medication. In December 1998 an independent research team evaluated the pilot and announced the results. The court-ordered group spent a median six weeks in the hospital while the non-coerced group spent fourteen. Over twice as many in the latter group were sent on for longer-term care to a state hospital. These results are even more impressive considering that patients in the court-ordered group were more likely to abuse drugs and alcohol, behavior that further increases the risk of hospitalization.[82]

In December 1998 the New York City Department of Mental Health held a hearing at Bellevue to help decide what would happen after the project's expiration in June 1999. A procession of consumer-survivor activists, including lawyers for rights groups like the Urban Justice Center, testified against outpatient commitment. Some of the witnesses were on the state payroll, employed as "peer specialists" by the Office of Mental Health; several were members of the Mental Patients Liberation Alliance, a group that also receives state funding. "Psychiatry kills," a frazzled young black woman from the Support Coalition warned the audience.[83] "We're living in Nazi Germany," she added. Then she played the race card:

> For a long time African Americans have been primary targets of the mental health system. Organizations like the National Alliance for the Mentally Ill, plus federal and state governments, are campaigning now to escalate psychiatric oppression of African Americans. A big part of this campaign is to increase the use of court orders and other coercion to force psychiatric drugs into people living out in the community itself, such as through legal orders called "involuntary outpatient commitment." This amounts to the government and the drug industry pushing drugs into the community.[84]

Although every one of the witnesses who actually had experience with the Bellevue pilot program (patients, their family members, staff) favored its continuation, nearly half of the forty-five witnesses spoke out against outpatient commitment. "Consumer-survivors and their advocates are swept up in denying the reality of mental illness," says Howard Telson, the psychiatrist who directed the Bellevue project.[85] "They blame the fact that patients don't take their medication on everything but the illness itself. Consumer-survivors misguidedly think that medication would be unnecessary if only the staff were more compassionate or provided more services." Yet, as Telson points out, and even some critics admit, the Bellevue project gave excellent services. And the fact remains that psychosis itself can make people resistant to taking medications. About one in two afflicted patients are so delusional, and their thinking so disordered, that they simply have no insight into the fact that they are ill.[86]

Despite the controversy surrounding the Bellevue project, Telson is a hero to the patients in his program and their families. Mel Silverman, whose forty-three-year-old son, a Cornell graduate, is a patient in the Bellevue project, testified at the hearings that he is the envy of other parents with mentally ill children. In Silverman's words: "My son is doing better now than he ever has during the last twenty-three years of his illness. You name the hospital in the New York City metro area, and he's been in it. He is now on an even keel for the first time in so long."

Roxanne Lanquetot also testified. "After our son refused to continue a new medication, we were frantic. He shrieked, laughed hysterically and stopped visiting us because the voices in his head forbad him to come up to the tenth floor, where the apartment is. [Now in the Bellevue program] we parents are relieved. Our son has not stopped taking medication nor decompensated since he was last in the hospital."

When patients, parents and clinicians spoke movingly about outpatient commitment—several proclaiming it "lifesaving"—many of the consumer-survivors in the audience booed and heckled them. When one of the patients left the podium after describing how much he had improved on the program, catcalls of "traitor" echoed through the auditorium.

Saving the Bellevue program took on added urgency when, three weeks after the hearings, thirty-two-year-old Kendra Webdale was pushed to her death under a Manhattan subway train. Andrew Goldstein, a man with schizophrenia who was about Webdale's age, was charged with the crime. Goldstein had been in and out of hospitals, halfway houses and clinics. Many times he himself asked to be admitted to the hospital. When he took medication, he was stable; when he stopped, he spiraled back into the abyss of psychosis.[87]

Out of Kendra Webdale's tragedy came two good things. The first was "Kendra's Law," passed by the New York legislature in the summer of 1999; it extended the Bellevue program and expanded outpatient commitment policies statewide. The second was Governor George Pataki's decision to impose a moratorium on hospital discharges and to put more money toward outpatient programs.[88] Predictably, consumer-survivors condemned the moratorium, insisting that only more outpatient services and residential facilities were needed. Granted, better outpatient care and housing are needed, but no matter how sophisticated and accommodating they are, these measures will never be enough for all patients. The protection of institutions and the oversight of Kendra's Law are critical for a small but potentially dangerous minority.

Yet Kendra's Law itself almost did not survive the consumers and the civil liberties bar. A key senator, Thomas Libous, chairman of the Senate Mental Health Committee, was set to vote against the bill, probably influenced in his decision by mental health "consumers," their legal advocates, advocates for the homeless and even some "soft on commitment" mental health professionals who testified before his committee.[89] In the end, Libous did vote for Kendra's Law, but I suspect that, like many politicians trying to balance a respect for civil rights with the need for legitimate paternalism, he was swayed by consumers' allegations that outpatient commitment was "torturous," "coercive" and "disproportionately aimed at people of color."[90]

The True Shame

In 1948 Albert Deutsch shocked the world with *Shame of the States,* his exposé of abuses in state psychiatric hospitals. The horrors he described have mostly disappeared, although newspapers still carry the occasional investigative account of abuses in a state facility.[91] In the dystopic worldview of the radical consumer-survivors, however, the mental health system remains a snake pit. Yet that very system provides the money with which they have financed a small industry of grievance and entitlement. It is the same hated system that has bent over backward to create places for consumer-survivors in its organizational charts. So much for oppression.

The point of imposing treatment is to help patients attain autonomy, to help them break out of the figurative straitjacket binding thought and will. So many people with untreated schizophrenia become incapable of facing even the modest challenges of ordinary life, much less exercising their rights as individuals. Being required to take medication is hardly a violation of the civil rights of a person who is too ill to exercise free will in the first place. The freedom to be psychotic is not freedom.

As a psychiatrist and a taxpayer, I find it a tragedy that consumer-survivors spend their time and energy—and public funds that could be going to patient care—fighting against policies that can help thousands who are far sicker than they are and, one hopes, will ever be. I realize that the political fight may itself be a form of therapy for consumer-survivors:

it gives them focus, identity and a social network. It funnels their energies and large reserves of anger. They are right to want a sense of purpose; we all need one. But the price of their "therapy" must not be paid by the very people they purport to protect.

I must also reserve criticism for the mental health administrators, some of whom are psychiatrists. Tragically, they seem willing to sacrifice the needs of those with the most severe illnesses to political correctness and to the expediency of placating the vocal and annoying consumer-survivor lobby. We have more effective treatments, both social and pharmacological, than ever in the history of psychiatry, and it is a shame when ill people are denied them. By supporting consumer-survivor activities—or by simply saying nothing when they are given funding or administrative control—mental health administrators are promoting a movement that has had disastrous consequences for people with severe psychiatric illness.

3

Nursing Grudges

In the summer of 1998 a group of nurses gathered at a university in New England for a graduate-level class. Just as the class was ending, a groundskeeper who had been working in the heat outdoors walked in and told the nurses he was feeling faint. Earlier in the week, he explained, he had suffered a hard blow to the head. Full of sympathy and concern, the nurses jumped into action.

Here is what these trained professionals did. Numerous pairs of hands began waving a few inches from the groundskeeper's body as the nurses assessed his "human energy field." One student told him that what he really needed was "a good cry." Finally, one nurse thought to put together the man's symptoms with his recent head trauma and suspected, correctly, that a blood clot was forming around his brain. The man required emergency medical attention to relieve the life-threatening condition.[1]

The quick-thinking student who rushed the groundskeeper off to the hospital was merely acting as any trained nurse would. The heart-stopping question is: What on earth were his classmates, all fellow nurses, doing?

The answer is "therapeutic touch," or TT. Developed in the 1970s by Dolores Krieger (no relation to Nancy Krieger), a professor of nursing at New York University, and her mentor Dora Kunz, TT draws on a theory of life force from Eastern religions and from the concept of animal magnetism postulated during the eighteenth century. Contrary to what its name suggests, TT (also called reiki) is not derived from the evangelical tradition of laying-on-of-hands practiced by faith healers. In fact, no hands ever touch the patient. Instead, practitioners sweep their hands over the patient to adjust the "human energy field" that supposedly surrounds and penetrates him. A freely flowing and symmetrical field is a prerequisite for health, practitioners claim, and by resolving energy blockages, TT can treat many problems, including high blood pressure, premenstrual cramps and lingering infections.

Although TT fails to pass objective tests of effectiveness, it is warmly embraced by the two most powerful nursing organizations in the country: the National League for Nursing and the American Nurses Association (ANA). The league accredits the nation's nursing colleges and actively promotes TT through books and videotapes. The ANA holds TT workshops at its national conventions, while the North American Nursing Diagnosis Association, a division of the ANA, explicitly recognizes "energy field disturbance" as a diagnosis—and the prescribed treatment is TT.[2] Indeed, the official publication of the ANA ran an article about "healing touch" with the teaser, "Take a closer look at one of the 'energetic' therapies. It just might recharge your practice."[3] TT has been the subject of numerous doctoral dissertations and master's theses written by advanced degree nurses.[4]

To stay updated, nurses can earn a continuing education certificate in TT through the American Holistic Nurses' Association, and practitioners can follow the "Standards of Care and Scope of Practice for Therapeutic Touch" and "Policy and Procedure for Health Professionals" published by the Nurse Healers–Professional Associates International.[5] In 1994 the ANA annual convention in San Antonio offered not only the traditional continuing education tracks but a "healing arts" track, which explored energy fields and TT and included the seminar "Crones, Nurses and Witches."[6] As the Colorado Board of Nursing has stated, "TT is completely within the mainstream of modern nursing practice."[7]

How can this be? Part of the answer is that these nurses share their fervor for TT with millions of other Americans who swear by unproven or discredited treatment techniques. But their TT campaign is also fueled by something else: a fiery resentment of the medical establishment, the so-called male medical elite.[8] Their antipathy represents a thoroughly postmodern rejection of the prevailing medical culture wherein doctors direct the patient's treatment and nurses carry out many of those directives. Here we see, once again, the drama of the dominant over the disenfranchised.

To stake out their own expertise in protest over physicians' "privileged" status and vast store of technical knowledge, postmodern nurses have decided to champion non-Western healing techniques, like TT. They have assailed researchers who question TT's effectiveness, accusing them of simply wanting to preserve control over medical practice in general, and over the predominantly female nursing profession in particular. In their journals, PC nurses challenge the very idea that medical knowledge should be obtained in an unbiased, repeatable and controlled fashion.

As we will see, these power struggles over therapeutic techniques and the conduct of clinical research are unhealthy for both patients and the nursing profession alike.

April Fools

On April 1, 1998, the nurses' good vibrations about TT were perturbed. The *Journal of the American Medical Association* published a paper demonstrating, quite literally, that TT is such quackery that even a child can debunk it.[9] The study undercut the idea behind TT by showing that its own practitioners could not reliably detect the presence of a human energy field. The authors recruited twenty-one TT practitioners and asked them to perceive the human energy field by putting their hands, palms up, through two cutouts at the base of a screen. On the other side of the screen, obscured from the practitioner's view, was the examiner, who held her right hand, palm down, about four inches above one of the practitioner's hands. Each practitioner underwent ten trials in which she was asked to detect whether the examiner's hand was positioned above her left or right hand. The result? The practitioners were no more likely to be correct than if they had simply guessed.

One of the paper's authors was nine-year-old Emily Rosa of Loveland, Colorado. She had devised the experiment for her fourth-grade science fair. The novelty of a child exposing a popular alternative therapy became a media sensation. Emily and her project got front-page coverage in the *New York Times* and the *Los Angeles Times*. She was featured in *Time* and *People* magazines and appeared on NBC's *Today Show*.

It is not difficult to imagine the reaction of the alternative medicine community. Susan B. Collins of the American Holistic Nurses Association said that she cared "very little whether a practitioner can feel energetic exchange in a contrived situation . . . when I see outcomes that the TT process as a whole works."[10] Mary Ireland of the Rutgers College of Nursing dismissed the experiment as unrealistic because, among other things, "it glosse[d] over the fact that practitioners generally use both hands to assess the Human Energy Field."[11] Cynthia Hutchinson, a TT instructor in Boulder, Colorado, with a doctorate in nursing, told the *Los Angeles Times* that *JAMA* itself was complicit because "it is a political organization and many physicians . . . feel threatened by human aura therapy because it means that their power and money are being taken away."[12] On Internet bulletin boards nurses scoffed at the work of a nine-year-old—never mind that the paper was stringently peer-reviewed, not by other nine-year-olds but by medical experts.[13]

Even Dr. Andrew Weil, the alternative medicine guru, weighed in. "I don't buy [Emily Rosa's] findings," he wrote in his "Ask Dr. Weil" online column. "There is too much evidence that healing energy systems work in cultures throughout the world, in a variety of forms."[14] Indeed, TT has multicultural appeal. According to the textbook *Nursing Diagnosis: Application to Clinical Practice*, TT helps us "celebrate the diversity among us. . . . Because of our Western culture orientation, we search for research to explain its effects. The Eastern mind doesn't care how it works, only that it does."[15] This is not so, of course. The practical Western mind happily exploits therapies that are effective even if it doesn't understand why. In fact, many mainstream therapies—lithium for manic-depression, morphine for pain, aspirin for stroke prevention—were used for years before anyone knew precisely how they worked. The problem with TT advocates is that so many of them resist demands to prove that their therapy works *at all.*

Emily Rosa's article in *JAMA* was a surgical strike against a movement that has gained impressive momentum. According to the National Council for Reliable Health Information, there are approximately fifty thousand practitioners of TT in this country today.[16] Therapeutic touch is offered in at least two hundred hospitals, including Columbia Presbyterian Hospital in New York City and Georgetown Medical Center in Washington, D.C. More than eighty university nursing colleges in North America teach TT elective courses. Most of the major hospitals of Denver and Boulder offer TT to patients. The Swedish Hospital in Denver even has a special "Department of Energy" (as in psychic energy). TT has also attracted federal tax money. The Division of Nursing of the Department of Health and Human Services gave a $200,000 grant to D'Youville Nursing Center in Buffalo, New York, to train student nurses in the technique. And the University of Alabama at Birmingham received $355,000 from the Department of Defense to study the use of TT to promote healing and pain relief in burn patients. The National Center for Nursing Research and the Office of Alternative Medicine, both at the National Institutes of Health, have made grants as well.[17]

What does TT look like? A typical TT session lasts between ten and thirty minutes; it is performed by a practitioner who first must be "centered"—a state of mind achievable through meditation. She scans the patient with hovering hands, searching for imbalances in the energy field, claiming to feel through her hands a sensation of tingling, throbbing or heat when they pass over areas of pain, inflammation or tension. Then she sweeps her hands over the patient in order to distribute excess energy to areas of deficit. If the practitioner thinks she has picked up excess or negative energy, she literally shakes it off her hands.

According to TT proponents, the technique can actually be dangerous if not performed properly. As Dolores Krieger, the mother of TT, writes, "Human energies are not well understood at this time, but we do know that indiscriminate and persistent interaction can overload the human system; a healee can overdose on human energies."[18] She also warns that if the healer is emotionally upset or physically ill, she can "transfer negative energy" to the patient, making him sicker. While this is no more plausible than TT itself, if the practitioner believes it, then she should inform the patient of this potential side effect. But many do not; TT is often performed without consent on patients who are asleep or in a coma, or on infants whose parents are unaware that their child is being "treated."

The Placebo Cure

Given the enthusiasm of TT promoters and their confidence in the procedure, one might imagine that a few of them would have tried to win the $1 million "Paranormal Challenge." The magician James Randi ("The Amazing Randi") offered the huge reward to anyone who could detect the human energy field. As of February 2000, Mr. Randi told me, only one person has taken the challenge since the offer was put on the table in 1998. And she failed.[19]

No surprise. Human energy fields don't exist. But the human condition does. Common sense tells us that a sick person who is frightened, lonely or bored will probably feel a bit better after receiving attention from a caring, unhurried individual. Or perhaps the patient experiences a "placebo effect": the illusion of having received an effective therapy. Generally we think of placebos as inactive ("sugar") pills, but they can also take the form of hand-waving. Research routinely shows that between 35 and 75 percent of patients experience relief if they believe they have been given an effective therapy for pain or anxiety. Thus, experimenters typically use a placebo in their research design so that they can be more confident that the effects of the new therapy they are testing exceed the "benefit" associated with placebo.

The promise of relief can be powerful. Sometimes even physical symptoms, not just subjective complaints like pain, nausea or mood, can improve after a patient receives a placebo. For example, the symptoms of full-blown heroin withdrawal—diarrhea, sweating, vomiting—can be reversed in some addicts simply by administering an injection of inert saline that they believe to be morphine. In surgery as well, patients have reported mild improvement of some neurological illnesses with placebo, or "sham," surgery in which the physician goes through all the preparations for surgery, including making the initial incisions in the skin, but does not actually operate on the brain.

Keep in mind, of course, that experimenters who have faith in the treatment they are testing can be as suggestible as the patients who want it to work. This means that both must be "blind" to whether the patient received the real or the sham therapy. An experimenter who knows which patients received the actual medication, for example, may inadvertently give them subtle hints about her confidence in the drug or her expectation that they will feel better. Even the surgeon performing a sham operation does not know whether she will perform the real surgery or simply make the skin incisions until she is in the operating room with the patient anesthetized.

It is very likely that TT recipients who feel better afterward are simply experiencing the time-honored placebo effect. This effect has rightly been called a window into the mind-body connection, but it is by no means a magical phenomenon. In fact, any number of not-so-mysterious processes can explain why some patients experience relief after taking a dummy pill. Sometimes it is as simple as self-deception.

A colleague of mine had a dramatic encounter with this. One of his patients with breast cancer had undergone a double mastectomy and chemotherapy, but her tumor returned, spreading to her chest wall, where it created obvious bumps under her skin. In desperation, she went to an offshore clinic for vitamin therapy and upon returning from the clinic a few weeks later saw my colleague again. She was a new woman, he said, buoyant, thrilled at her medical progress. "My tumors have disappeared," she told him, "look for yourself." But when he unwrapped the bandages on her chest, he saw that not only were the tumorous nodules still present, but they had become infected and were literally crawling with maggots. The woman died a week later.[20]

If some people can fool themselves about remission of major diseases, imagine the possibilities for perceiving that minor ailments have diminished.

Placebo effects do not always represent self-deception, of course. Sometimes improvement is real, most likely owing to the complex relationship between mental state and the immune, cardiovascular and hormonal systems. This is why many researchers agree on the need for investigations into the placebo effect itself, its duration, the conditions under which it seems to manifest and the ethics of its application. Through such work we may learn more about the psychology, physiology and control of pain. Until we know more, it is reasonable to theorize that a patient who is reassured by the practitioner and confident of feeling better may undergo some physiological changes, such as endorphin release, heart-rate decline and lower levels of stress hormones like corticosteroid.

How long these physiological changes last and how dramatic they are vary from person to person. Although they rarely alter the course of serious illness, they can explain much of the benign effects associated with placebo. Conversely, placebos can also produce ill effects (the so-called nocebo effect). When patients are told that they may experience annoying side effects like tingling, nausea or headache after taking a pill, many will indeed report such symptoms. Presumably the body produces these symptoms in response to suggestion, even though it was a dummy pill that was taken.

What's the Harm in TT?

What is wrong with indulging our fascination with the mystical and occult? This is a question asked by Dr. Marcia Angell in her 1996 book *Science on Trial: The Clash of Medical Evidence and the Law in the Breast Implant Case.* Nothing . . . until we start deceiving ourselves. The "disdain for science has vast implications for how we come to know the truth about the human body," Angell writes. The topic of her book is silicone breast implant litigation (a saga of lawyers and patients claiming implant-induced illness where science could find none), but her message applies to alternative medicine (a saga of practitioners and patients claiming healing—from, say, TT—where there really isn't any). As the physicist Robert Park sums it up: "Alternative seems to define a culture rather than a field of medicine—a culture that is not scientifically demanding."[21]

Nonetheless, alternative medicine is popular. According to the director of the Center for Complementary and Alternative Medicine at NIH, 42 percent of all Americans used one or more alternative treatments in 1997, up from one-third in 1991.[22] This is understandable. Alternative practitioners are known for spending more time with patients than mainstream doctors. Moreover, many of the interventions appear effective—I say "appear" because, in many instances, either the problem would have gone away on its own or it may have responded to the placebo effect.

Lastly, some people turn to alternative approaches when mainstream medicine has run out of answers. The clinic of a practitioner who is enthusiastic about his treatments, generous with his time and full of promises about relief or even cure can seem an irresistible oasis of hope. The downside, however, can be devastating. As the anthropologist and physician Melvin Konner writes: "Some take herbs with serious but completely unstudied adverse effects. Some empty their bank accounts and give up their last months with their families to travel from one healer to the next, trying untested therapies and changing their faiths like overcoats in an effort to fend off pain and fear."[23]

Despite these dangers—indeed, *because* of these dangers—doctors must keep up with the unconventional therapies their patients may be using. It is crucial for physicians and advanced practice nurses to be familiar with the range of herbs, natural food store items, Eastern interventions like acupuncture and so on. Doctors should be prepared to answer questions ("Does Saint-John's-wort really help with depression?") and know which novel therapies are showing promise in well-designed clinical trials. They should know the risks involved in fad diets and which alternative treatments can be dangerous if combined with conventional medical treatment. They should be ready to prevent needless tragedies that can arise when sick people waste time on fad therapies before turning to conventional treatment, or when they substitute an alternative treatment altogether.

Most medical schools now offer instruction in alternative medicine, either full courses or a series of lectures. But teaching about alternative medicine should not be a license to advocate for it uncritically. According to a review in *Academic Medicine* by Dr. Wallace Sampson of the Stanford University School of Medicine, a worrisome fraction of the course instructors are quite partisan about alternative medicine, extolling its virtues despite lack of data.[24] When Sampson asked about their teaching philosophy, a number of course directors had some pretty shaky responses. The one who exposed students to past lives therapy (a form of "therapy" that helps you discover who you were in, say, the Middle Ages) did so in order "to open the door of possibility." Others spoke of not being "judgmental" ("We believe in the First Amendment," said one director). "Healing is about love," said a course description.

The University of Chicago, by contrast, is approaching alternative medicine responsibly. Recently the university's medical school received a $5 million grant from the Tang Foundation to study the effects of Chinese herbs that have been used for centuries in the East and are gaining popularity in the United States. "The most important thing is to make discoveries," said Professor Shutsung Liao, a biochemist who will oversee the research.[25] Indeed, discovery, not dogmatic faith in unproven methods, is how medical schools and nursing schools should approach the subject of alternative medicine.

Florence Nightingale Meets Gloria Steinem

To some extent, nurses' efforts to set themselves apart from mainstream medicine by practicing and extolling TT reflect a jockeying for turf that occurs regularly between related professions. Nurse anesthetists, for example, have tried for years to loosen the requirement that anesthesiologists supervise them; nurse practitioners and physicians have tussled over the extent of the former's authority to prescribe drugs.[26]

But feminism has imbued some nurses with an ideological zeal that goes far beyond guild issues. "Women nurses are women first," writes the nurse Jo Ann Ashley in her article "Power Is Structured Misogyny," which appeared in the journal *Advances in Nursing Sciences*. Instead of complementing the doctor's traditional "curing" role with their traditional "caring" role, some nurses are pitting care against cure.[27] They bristle at the

Florence Nightingale image of the nurse as a woman obedient to the doctor—his "handmaiden," as Nightingale put it. Postmodern nurses would rather fly the banner of victimhood unfurled in the 1970s by feminists like Barbara Ehrenreich and Deirdre English, who wrote in their pamphlet *Witches, Midwives and Nurses:*

> Our oppression as women health workers today is inextricably linked to our oppression as women. Nursing, our predominant role in the health system, is simply a workplace extension of our roles as wife and mother. The nurse is socialized to believe that rebellion violates not only her "professionalism," but her very femininity. This means the male medical elite has a very special stake in the maintenance of sexism in the society at large: Doctors are the bosses in an industry where the workers are primarily women. . . . Take away sexism and you take away one of the mainstays of the health hierarchy.[28]

Kathryn A. Ballou, a clinical instructor in nursing at the University of Missouri (and practicing indoctrinologist), finds herself immersed in nursing's struggle for recognition and autonomy. If nurses truly wish to advance "our professional power base," she exclaims, they will need to liberate themselves from the confines of the medical profession. "Imitation of an oppressor group such as medicine will only keep us oppressed," Ballou contends. "Otherwise we will most assuredly continue to feel unappreciated and powerless."[29]

Adeline R. Falk Rafael of the University of Colorado School of Nursing complains that simply being female has consigned women to the nursing profession. Femininity has prepared women to be dominated, she contends, making them submissive, helpless, dependent, nurturing and altruistic. "Even today," Rafael laments, "nurses' language suggests [that] deference is still required of nurses as they follow 'orders' that physicians write."[30] In describing the nurse-physician relationship, a Canadian nurse named A. J. Baumgart says that nurses, like women everywhere, are denied "rightful knower status." In a patriarchal system, as Baumgart describes it, the nurse "should not know" because knowledge is the province of the (male) physician.[31]

All this talk of oppression ignores the remarkable progress women have made in medicine. With women accounting for about half of all health administrators and almost half of all medical students, the medical establishment is no longer overwhelmingly male. Nurses can now train for jobs with considerable clinical responsibility, like advanced practice nursing, with a salary range of $55,000 to 75,000 per year, depending on experience and location. An advanced practice nurse can prescribe many types of medications and order and interpret laboratory tests. Nurse midwives can deliver babies. Nurses in neonatal, coronary and surgical intensive-care units track vital signs, clean and monitor invasive catheters, evaluate heart monitor readouts and manage fragile metabolic states. Nursing has come a very long way since the days of Florence Nightingale.

Women's Studies Goes to Nursing School

Indoctrinologist nurses have retaliated against doctors' alleged monopoly on clinical knowledge by creating their own literature. It contains heavy doses of polemic and social criticism, as exemplified by the work of Jean Watson, a professor in the University of Colorado School of Nursing and former president of the National League of Nursing. As Watson writes in the *Nursing Science Quarterly:*

> Postmodern directions are already evident in nursing science knowledge and contemporary nursing theories. . . . This shift in extant nursing science and knowledge matrix is reflected in such shared concepts as evolution of consciousness, self-transcendence, open system, harmony, relativity of space-time, patterning, and holism. . . . In summary, as nursing locates itself within the postmodern condition of complexity, with its shadow and light side, and as nursing seeks a dwelling place which is open-ended, ambiguous, dynamically constructed, incessantly questioned, endlessly self-revising, never set, but floating and moving with the river of life, will nurses be part of helping nursing to mature and grow up both ontologically and epistemologically, within its own transformative praxis paradigm?[32]

Confused? Watson's paper calls to mind the 1996 Alan Sokal affair. Sokal was a physics professor who published a paper in *Social Text,* an influential academic journal of cultural studies, in which he argued absurdly that gravity is a social construct with no objective reality. But while Sokal's paper was a brilliant hoax, Watson means for hers to be taken seriously. And her work is not unusual. Publications such as the *Journal of Transcultural Nursing, Advances in Nursing Science,* the *Journal of Nursing Education* and *Nursing Inquiry* are brimming with incomprehensible sentences that create the illusion of scholarship:

- From "Nursing the Postmodern Body" in *Nursing Inquiry:* "Using touch as a medium for exploring the ways in which it is constructed by nurses, the body is here characterized by a plethora of competing and co-existing terms: disobedient, obedient, mirroring, stigmatized, sinful, post-mortem . . . dominant, dominating, deceitful, disciplined, postmodern and communicative."[33]

- From "Global Migration and Health: Ecofeminist Perspectives" in *Advances in Nursing Science:* "[Ecofeminism is] the parallel oppression and domination of women and nature originating from a single logic of domination."[34]

- From "Understanding Women's Risk of HIV Infection in Thailand Through Critical Hermeneutics" in *Advances in Nursing Science:* "Women's oppression in Thailand is discussed as a position made of the moral imperative to use counterhegemonic methodologies in the study of HIV risk and prevention."[35]

- From "Correlates of Prejudice in Nursing Students" in the *Journal of Nursing Education:* "Most health workers are socialized in the 'equal treatment' model, that all patients/clients should be treated exactly the same. This equal treatment model emerges from a Eurocentric, middle class perspective and often takes a paternalistic, patronizing view of the diverse patient/client as a child in need of protection and guidance."[36]

- From "Inquiry into the Paranormal" in *Nursing Science Quarterly:* "Research of the paranormal may provide the theoretical base for the spontaneous remission of cancer. It is feasible that the rhythmical waves of paranormal manifestation can participate in patterning blood pressure, heart rate, and the flow of substances such as insulin. This might lessen dependence upon external substances such as medication. Undoubtedly there would be great savings for the health care system and many drug companies might go bankrupt."[37]

The health journalist Sarah Glazer has waded through the post-structural nursing narratives and observes: "For these nurses, words like 'reality,' 'objectivity,' 'evidence-based practice,' 'quantitative research,' and even 'measurement' have become code words for all that is evil, patriarchal, and insensitive about modern medicine and modern science."[38]

Sometimes nursing "scholarship" lapses into New Age sentimentality. Consider this poem by a nurse midwife cited, approvingly, in the *Nursing Science Quarterly:*

> *And when it comes I examine the placenta*
> *I'm sorting the particles and waves in the spectrum of light*
> *And when my work is finished I go from the place of birth*
> *I walk out across the fields of the planets into the spaces between*
>   *the furthest stars.*[39]

Gail J. Mitchell of the University of Toronto brushes aside the quest for scientific evidence. The "professional nursing practice is a living, unfolding mutuality of inter-subjective being with," she says. "What, then, can come from research findings that are generalized from persons not present in the nurse-person process?"[40] Quite a bit. One need not be immersed in the "nurse-person process" to generate important findings about nursing practice.

Julie Sochalski of the Center for Health Outcomes at the University of Pennsylvania School of Nursing is conducting research "that is giving us insight into scores of important issues, like the relationship between staffing patterns and patient outcome; how to predict which premature babies are at greatest risk; how hospitals can retain good nurses (answer: give them greater measures of autonomy); which pain guidelines are most effective and easiest for the nurse to follow."[41] Sochalski and her colleagues at the University of Pennsylvania are by no means a vanishing species, but the thorough absence of rigorous and empirical analysis from much of the nursing literature has a number of academic nurses rightly concerned. "I find I reject over 90 percent of the manuscripts I am sent as a peer reviewer for scholarly journals," Mark Avis of England's School of Nursing at the University of Nottingham tells me. "I am also appalled by the poor standards of reviewing amongst my peers and horrified by the poor scholarship of some of the papers that do get accepted."[42] Little surprise, then, that nursing was the lowest-rated of the seventy-two scholarly subjects examined in the 1992 Research Selectivity Exercise conducted by the Universities Funding Council of the United Kingdom.[43]

Lorraine N. Smith, a professor of nursing at the University of Glasgow, compared three influential nursing journals to the *British Medical Journal*. She found that the studies published in the nursing journals had much smaller sample sizes and were sometimes missing vital information, such as whether samples were randomly chosen or what kinds of statistical analyses were used. "Nursing research is in danger of being seen as possessing much rhetoric and little substance," Smith writes.[44]

The problem is not limited to British nursing. Writes Susan R. Gortner, a professor of nursing at the University of California at San Francisco, "Empiricism has been given short shrift in nursing." It has, she says, been "criticized for the very features that have made it the mainstay of scientific work . . . precision, caution, and skepticism about outcomes."[45] Barbara J. Drew, a coronary-care nurse in a San Francisco hospital, makes a "plea not to devalue the biological sciences at a time when a majority of nurses are drawing heavily from biological knowledge to provide increasingly complex care" to sicker patients. She adds: "In recoiling from the male-dominated, reductionist, disease-oriented biomedical model, nursing science has (perhaps unintentionally) narrowed its scope primarily to study the social and behavioral sciences."[46]

Postmodernism may be a harmless approach to literary criticism, but in medicine the stakes are much higher. A health professional who brings the concept of relativism to her work is a frightening prospect. If she does not see the importance of making judgments about and distinctions between treatments, she will lead patients to make bad decisions—say, choosing a homeopathic remedy (basically water) over radiation or chemotherapy for a treatable cancer. "This is not the Enlightenment triumph of autonomous persons resolving problems using objective standards of evidence, reason, and logic," contends Donal P. O'Mathuna of the Mount Carmel College of Nursing. "It is the postmodern triumph of individuals creating their own truths because no objective truth exists."[47]

At Least Do No Harm

How is PC nursing manifested in the real world? Ask Kevin Courcey, a nurse at Sacred Heart Medical Center in Eugene, Oregon. In April 1998, Courcey was one of millions to read about Emily Rosa's TT experiment in the local paper. He was elated: "Finally someone had figured out how to call the bluff of TT practitioners."[48] The next week a colleague of Courcey's who is a surgical nurse told him of a strange experience. The nurse, who has asked me to call her "Helen" for fear of losing her job at Sacred Heart if identified, had been attending a postoperative patient. She left the room for a moment to get some pain medication. When she returned, another hospital staff member was at the bedside and told Helen that she "could help take away the patient's pain with therapeutic touch" and that no medication was needed. Helen watched as her colleague proceeded to wave her hands over the patient as though capturing the pain with her hands and shaking it off at the foot of the bed. After a few minutes the patient said that her pain had indeed diminished. Distracted by the dramatic, sweeping gestures, the patient did not notice, until Helen pointed it out, that she had just been given IV pain medication. "I was concerned that if the patient hadn't been informed about the pain medication, she would have attributed her relief to the magical arm-waving," Helen says. "I felt this would have constituted fraudulent medical practice."

Later that week Courcey noticed that Sacred Heart was offering two TT courses for staff nurses, one for beginners and one for those who had been practicing for at least six months and who "felt ready to deepen their sensitivities and awareness of their practice." Why, he wondered, was a modern hospital not only permitting worthless therapy but also training even more nurses to do it? Perturbed, Courcey took these questions to the medical chief of staff at Sacred Heart. The chief expressed concern, but nothing happened. "As nurses, we are held responsible by the state Nurse Practice Act to protect patients and report malpractice," Courcey tells me. TT, he says, is "malpractice." Indeed, the ANA "Code for Nurses" states that "the nurse participates in the profession's efforts to protect the public from misinformation and misrepresentation."[49]

The Questionable Nursing Practices Task Force of the National Council for Reliable Health Information keeps track of such nursing misadventures.[50] Here are some cases from its files:

- A man in much pain was asked by a nurse whether he would "like some help with relaxation techniques." Instead of reporting the unusual amount of pain to the physician, the nurse sent in an aide to do "healing touch." When he saw her waving her hands over him, he thought he was getting his last rites and became panicked.

- In another case, a patient was so startled by the hand-waving of a TT practitioner that he fell out of bed and broke his arm.

- A woman with abdominal pain went to a TT nurse who had a private practice. The nurse recommended TT treatments only, and the woman died of complications from a ruptured appendix a few days later.

- A woman who called her HMO nurse on-call when she developed severe abdominal pain was told that she should use the pain to get in touch with her inner self. Nothing else. The woman went to an emergency room, where she was found to have a pelvic mass, later determined to be a large ovarian tumor.

Some nurses report being pressured to perform TT. When Elaine Bishop, an oncology nurse, was instructed to participate in TT training by nursing administration at a hospital in Grand Rapids, Michigan, she complained to an internal review committee of doctors and got TT banned from her hospital. "The doctors were easy to convince," Bishop recalls, "but the chief of nursing was another story. She wasn't pleased, to say the least."[51]

Sharon Fish, a community health nurse, found TT spiritually offensive. According to Fish, Christians cannot engage in TT without compromising their faith. As she reminds her colleagues, "[God] alone can teach the true meaning of the laying on of hands to comfort, care and cure."[52] Worse, for Fish, is that the neopagan Wiccan religion promotes a variant of TT—one major difference being that the Wiccan healer is nude when she manipulates life forces. Prompted by complaints from nurses who felt that their religious convictions were violated by hospital-sanctioned TT, the Equal Employment Opportunity Commission declared in 1988 that health care employees cannot be required to learn or practice TT.[53]

An Antiscience Agenda

What TT advocates lack in familiarity with scientific method they make up for in political savvy, as this story from the University of Colorado shows.

In 1994 a group of Colorado residents protested the use of taxpayer money to teach TT at the University of Colorado's Center for Human Caring. The university convened a panel of in-house and invited faculty members to review the scientific evidence for TT. Henry Claman, a professor of medicine and immunology at the university's medical school, led the panel, which found no evidence confirming TT's usefulness.[54]

Claman, a strong supporter of research, suggested to the nurses that they collaborate with energy scientists in the university's engineering department to study the hypothesized mechanism of TT. His offer went ignored, and in the end the nurses prevailed. Remarkably, the university turned the issue into a matter of academic freedom. "The university officials believed that removing the subject from the curriculum would violate the academic freedom of the nursing school," Claman has explained to me.[55] "There was no question that [the nurses] had an anti-male and anti-M.D. agenda," he said to Gina Kolata of the *New York Times*, "but they cleverly turned it into an issue of academic rights."[56]

The University of Texas School of Nursing is another institution that exercises its freedom to mislead students. The school's 1998–99 continuing education series for nurses, which was approved by the Texas State Board of Nursing and the American Nurses Credentialing Center Commission on Accreditation, includes such New Age offerings as "Using Energy to Enhance Nursing Practice: Use of Color, Music, Touch and Movement," "Holistic Nursing: Strategies That Transform and Heal," "Aromatherapy for Nursing Practice," "Reflexology: Stimulating Healing in the Body," "Spirituality in Nursing" and "Using the Power of Our Thoughts for Healing." Courses in herbal medicine and homeopathy are offered side by side with staples like poison control and pharmacology.[57]

These courses hardly seem consistent with the mission of the nursing school's continuing education department: to "harness the technological advances of the information age and help tomorrow's practicing nurses stay ahead." Stephen Barrett, a retired psychiatrist who is now a full-time chronicler of medical fads, is bemused. "Instead of creating an authentic program to enhance nurses as professionals, they are selling an antitechnology, antiscience, antidoctor agenda," he says.[58]

The University of Texas Skeptical Society was also appalled at the direction the curriculum was taking. Roahn H. Wynar, a graduate student in physics and society member, wrote a letter from the society in the spring of 1998 to all nursing school faculty members: "Help us [get] the Texas State Board of Nursing to get TT de-certified for continuing education credit," the letter said. "The researcher inside you must understand the silliness of TT as taught at UTSON. Why let this go on? Can we trust the work done at a school that collects money for quackery?"[59] Wynar was referring to the fee that nurses must pay to take continuing education courses. According to Wynar, everyone right on up to the university provost and the nursing school credentialing authority responded to this appeal by saying "everything was okay."

Starched Cap Blues

Conditions across the Atlantic provide an intriguing parallel to developments here. Thirty years ago British nurses were expected to observe rules of silence, ritual and courtesy. They were barred from getting married while in training, personal jewelry was banned and hair could not be longer than shoulder-length. Nurses were supervised by a strict ward matron who handed down orders. "I don't think anyone would like to see a complete return to the way things were," writes Minette Marrin, a *London Telegraph* columnist, "the ferocious matrons, the virginal seclusion of nurses' [dormitories], extreme deference to doctors . . . the starched cap." But, she says, British nursing has now embraced the opposite extreme.[60]

Other writers agree. In their essay "Extinguishing the Lamp," Janet Warren and Myles Harris note that "the nursing profession in England became stridently combative, 'rights based' and feminist. Nursing began to be billed as a wider struggle for better consumer rights, equality for minorities, 'gays,' any group which could be used as a means of exerting leverage for more pay and a 'better' image."[61] By 1995 all the traditional nursing schools had closed. Nursing training was expanded to include sociology, politics and race and gender awareness. Patient care suffered. The *Telegraph*'s Marrin cites the opinion of one National League of Nursing manager: young nurses, who often begin their careers unable to insert a catheter or to take blood pressure, are now "a liability on the wards."

Part of the problem is financial. "There is no doubt that many health managers would much prefer to see fewer expensively-trained nurses and far larger numbers of unskilled workers in the health service," Warren and Miles write. Thus, two trends—government efforts to cut costs and nurses' efforts to break out of the traditional nurse-doctor relationship—have combined to estrange nurses from the bedside. Unfortunately, patients tend to suffer when competent nurses are removed from the front lines of clinical work and the basics of practical nursing are left to orderlies and superficially trained health workers.

England now has a major crisis in nursing recruitment. From 1987 until 1994 the number of young women entering training fell 39 percent. The educational quality of applicants has also deteriorated, and dropout rates from nursing school are estimated at 15 to 20 percent over the course of the standard three-year training period. According to the Department of Education, some nurses are so weak in mathematics that they have difficulty calculating safe drug dosages.[62]

According to John Clare, education editor of the *Telegraph,* the literacy and numeracy skills of half of all British adults are so poor that they cannot cope with the demands of everyday life. Clare singles out nurses in his otherwise general report of a recently released European survey on literacy: "Nurses could be putting patients' lives at risk because poor standards in maths may lead to errors in calculating doses, it has been claimed. A meeting of the [nursing] profession's regulatory body, the United Kingdom Central Council for Nursing, was told that maths was a general weakness in nursing education."[63]

The situation in this country is not so dire, though it is worsening. Though the United States has more nurses in practice than ever—about 2.1 million in 1996, the most recent year for which there are government figures—there is a growing shortage of hospital nurses.[64] Nursing shortages per se are nothing new; they tend to occur in roughly ten-year cycles, according to Maryann F. Fralic, a professor at Johns Hopkins University School of Nursing. For a number of reasons, however, this one is different, and Fralic worries we may not be able to bounce back as reliably this time.[65]

One important dynamic driving the current shortage is the push to save money on hospital costs. Inpatient stays are shorter, beds are closing and more care is being delivered outside of the hospital. One consequence is that nurses have other work opportunities, such as providing home health care or doing utilization reviews for managed care companies. But another result is that the nurses who stay in the hospital setting are being worked to the bone. Marge Bradley of North Haven, Connecticut, is simply burned out: "I now have to delegate most tasks [of bedside care]. . . . More time is spent on the phone and at the computers than in [patients'] rooms. I have never given worse care in my life. I am a darn good nurse and I will leave before that changes."[66]

With higher thresholds for hospitalizing patients, fewer nurses care for sicker patients. In 1999 California became the first state to mandate ratios of nurses to patients in response to concerns that nurses are stretched to the breaking point and patient care is at risk.[67]

Another reason for declining enrollments in nursing schools is that women have far wider career options than ever before, both in medicine and in other professions. Claire Fagin, a former dean of the University of Pennsylvania's nursing school, says the recruitment problem will worsen "if women and men are encouraged to abandon caring roles in favor of more powerful and economically rewarding roles."[68] Also, during the mid-1990s, when managed care exploded, there was a general perception that staffing needs would favor unlicensed staff over more expensive and highly trained nurses. "It was discouraging to young women and men considering a nursing career," Fralic said. "They didn't want to go to nursing school if they had reason to think there would be fewer jobs for them."

According to the American Association of Colleges of Nursing, the number of enrollees in bachelor's and master's level nursing programs dropped 5.5 percent in 1998, the fourth straight decline. A spokeswoman for Samuel Merritt Nursing College in Oakland, California, told the *New York Times* in 1999 that the only way to keep college enrollment steady was to accept less-qualified applicants.[69] Thus, because of declining enrollment, the aging of the nursing workforce and the exodus from hospital to non-inpatient settings, when experienced nurses retire from acute-care settings like emergency rooms, operating rooms and intensive-care units, they are not being replaced fast enough. If current trends continue, estimate Peter Buerhaus of the Vanderbilt University School of Nursing and his colleagues, the nursing workforce will decline nearly 20 percent below projected requirements by the year 2020.[70]

Nursing Shortage and Affirmative Action

Compounding the nursing shortages is the problem of lowered academic standards in some nursing schools. Driven partly by the desperate need to recruit more nursing students and by an embrace of affirmative action, many schools are graduating young trainees who are poorly prepared.

This trend could not come at a worse time: with hospitals admitting only the sickest patients, nurses must be astute enough and cool enough under pressure to spot acute clinical changes and make quick decisions.

In California especially, the nursing shortage and affirmative action in nursing school admissions have combined to worrisome effect. Beginning in 1995, according to the *Los Angeles Times,* state nursing programs offered by community colleges have been mandated to adopt either "discrimination-proof" admission systems based on lotteries or first-come-first-served waiting lists made up of students with at least a C average in prerequisite courses.[71] Students with higher grades are turned away in order to ensure diversity.

The lack of selectivity has had alarming consequences. Some students are being held back because their accents are too heavy and can't be understood by patients. Several of the college instructors interviewed by the *Los Angeles Times* said that their students were stumped by the kind of single-variable algebra problem used to calculate drug dosages. "They can't read at a high school level . . . or they have undiagnosed learning disabilities," said Sue Albert, interim dean of Antelope Valley College.

As a result of taking any student with a C minimum, dropout rates in California schools have soared. Before the new admissions policy, about 5 percent of students did not complete the two-year nursing program. Now that rate has doubled, and some schools have reached a rate of two dropouts for every five enrollees. Grades have dropped, scores on the statewide nursing board exams have gone down as well and the number of students who need more than two years to finish their coursework has increased. Julie Herda, a pediatric nurse practitioner in Orange County, was moved to speak about the erosion of standards: "If indeed the California community college system cannot admit potential nursing candidates based on academic performance (as is the standard for other professions), the education of registered nurses does not belong in that [system]."[72]

In October 1999 a group of nursing instructors called for a meeting with Thomas Nussbaum, the community college chancellor. He decided to create a task force to develop more stringent nursing admission standards. Meanwhile, most nursing programs have been trying to repair the damage with intensive tutoring. While the 1995 mandate did allow for programs to set their own admissions standards, the catch was that they had to show that those standards would correlate with success. To date only a handful of programs have undertaken these efforts.

Mary Parker, head of nursing at Cuesta Community College in San Luis Obispo, told the *Los Angeles Times* that some students who were flunking out had expressed "suicidal" feelings in her office. Such desperate responses were not the norm, but there is little question that many students were falsely promised a chance at becoming a nurse. One wonders how quickly nursing education standards will be restored with groups like the National Organization of Nurse Practitioner Faculties bemoaning "power differentials." How can they be expected to confront students about their deficiencies when they themselves seem so confused about the legitimacy of academic paternalism? "What are the power and status discrepancies that we must work with before we can be effective teachers?" the organization asks its members, noting that "students are fearful of our power to grade."[73]

Who's Watching the Monitor?

"Therapeutic touch and alternative medicine have spread because a lot of good nursing academics have said nothing," says Linda Rosa, Emily Rosa's mother and herself a nurse. It isn't safe to merely assume that common sense will prevail, that the postmodernists will shrink in number and influence. Dumbing down the curriculum, teaching pseudo-science and promoting feel-good, unproven remedies are deeply worrisome trends. So is the flourishing of an orthodoxy that shuts out dissenting voices. Linda Rosa was told by a former editor of the *American Journal of Nursing*, the official publication of the American Nurses Association, that he would not publish anything critical of TT because "it would confuse" the readers.[74]

Responsible nurses owe it to their profession and to their patients to protest. "They must not tolerate the violation of students' trust when they see a colleague teaching TT (or homeopathy or crystal healing and so on) as a proven remedy," Rosa insists. Nursing schools, nursing journals, the American Nurses Association and the National League of Nursing should be taking the lead in applying critical judgment and scientific rigor and in rooting out the indoctrinologists among them. As Linda Rosa says, "Patients shouldn't have to wonder whether someone is watching their monitor or trying to balance their energy fields."

4

Sisterhood and Medicine

THE TOXICITY OF WOMEN'S BREASTS, according to Patricia Ireland, president of the National Organization for Women (NOW), will be one of the major political issues of the new millennium. In the fall of 1999 Ireland gathered on Capitol Hill with Representative Nancy Pelosi, the California Democrat, and leaders of the San Francisco–based Breast Cancer Fund and other advocacy groups to announce the formation of the National Breast Cancer Prevention Campaign.[1]

"There are hundreds of synthetic chemicals in breast milk," according to Ireland. "We are poisoning the earth, and women are dying because of it." Andrea Martin of the Breast Cancer Fund told the audience that rates of breast cancer are increasing. "We have a right to know what chemicals we are carrying around in our breast," she said. At the event, Ireland, Martin and the national campaign—which comprises about sixty women's and health advocacy organizations—demanded more federal funding for research into the role of a particular class of synthetic chemicals called "endocrine disrupters." Supposedly these chemicals interfere with human hormones (specifically estrogens) to cause a range of defects. "The evidence—and our bodies—continue to pile up," claim the advocates.[2]

Now for the facts. First, the death rate from breast cancer has been declining since the mid-1980s, according to the National Cancer Institute (NCI).[3] The incidence is increasing only for the less advanced stages of the disease.[4] This suggests that more women are being screened and that cancer detection is increasing as the quality and availability of mammography improves. Increased incidence need not mean that more new cases of cancer are cropping up. There can be a higher incidence because cases are detected earlier and thus patients who are diagnosed are staying alive—that's good news.

Second, the "endocrine disrupter" hypothesis trumpeted in a 1996 best-seller, *Our Stolen Future,* is scientifically bankrupt.[5] According to the book, estrogen-like substances found in man-made materials from plastics to pesticides are causing a host of problems, like infertility and breast cancer in humans and deformities in the sex organs of animals. While it is true that exposure to high levels of estrogen is a risk factor for breast and uterine cancers, and also that some man-made chemicals have weak estrogen-like effects, the authors of *Our Stolen Future* take a huge leap. They claim that these chemicals combine synergistically to produce a powerful estrogen-like effect that wreaks physiological havoc on our reproductive systems by disrupting the function of our own naturally produced estrogen. So alarmed was Congress by this claim that in 1996 it required the Environmental Protection Agency (EPA) to develop testing and screening guidelines for endocrine disrupters.

A closer look at the science, however, reveals numerous holes in this tapestry of doom. First, there are naturally occurring estrogenic compounds in fruits, nuts and vegetables that are far more potent in their estrogen-like effect than synthetic chemicals, yet the former are not considered risk factors for breast cancer. Second, the researchers at Tulane University who claimed in 1996 to have measured a strong estrogen-mimicking effect from synthetic chemicals retracted their own data a year later because their results could not be replicated.[6] Third, the environmental levels of most of the compounds suspected of being endocrine disrupters have decreased over the last few decades as a consequence of strict regulations regarding their use and disposal.[7]

Researching preventable causes of breast cancer is logical enough, but the National Breast Cancer Prevention Campaign's preoccupation with the role of man-made estrogenic chemicals in causing cancer is a triumph of junk science—that is, the promulgation of a cause-and-effect relationship where none has been shown to exist. As Jennifer R. Myhre of the sociology department of the University of California at Davis writes in the *Journal of the American Medical Women's Association:* "Regardless of the scientific merit of the claims that environmental pollution causes breast cancer, the growing interest in environmental issues among breast cancer activists is significant because it highlights the [breast cancer] movement's attempt to reframe breast cancer as a social issue."[8]

Promoting women's "social issues" through pseudo-science does not help women. It creates needless worry about health, takes women's focus away from actual risks and misdirects resources better spent on more promising avenues of research. Back in the 1970s the landscape was different. American women were more than ready for their own health movement. There was a growing intolerance of "our mother's gynecologist," who often possessed a patronizing, there-there-it's-all-in-your-head-little-lady attitude. Women wanted control of their physiology beyond contraception. They wanted more information, and they wanted doctors who let them ask questions.

The legitimate concerns and can-do spirit of the 1970s women's health movement have given way to a campaign largely fueled by misplaced aggrievement and misinformation. Many advocates claim—wrongly—that the medical establishment is still run by men, that the research enterprise is denying women medical breakthroughs and that neither is paying serious attention to women's medical needs.

Women's Bodies, Women's Fantasies

I recently happened upon an hour-long special on PBS featuring Christiane Northrup, a physician and author of the best-selling *Women's Bodies, Women's Wisdom: Creating Physical and Emotional Health and Healing.* Like the guru-doctors Deepak Chopra and Andrew Weil, who preceded her on public television as subjects of their own specials, Northrup spoke of "chakra energy," "cleansing" and "inner guidance." Here is a small sample of what she preaches:

- Aggressive behavior can be associated with cancer.

- An individual's perception of whether her body is permeable to influences, either physical or emotional, is related to whether she is susceptible to cancer.

- An overdeveloped will (overassertiveness) can result in hyperthyroidism.

- Blood clot formation is related to stopping the flow of intuitive information.[9]

Northrup is more than just another New Age physician; she is an expert in *women's* health. Strange, then, that some of the medical wisdom she dispenses is reminiscent of attitudes from one hundred years ago. (I say "some" of her wisdom because Northrup's discussion on the relative safety of breast implants, for example, is accurate, timely and thoughtful.) What the doctor is basically suggesting in much of her book sounds like a modern parody of Sigmund Freud: in other words, women are hysterics. As Freud described them in his 1895 classic *Studies on Hysteria*, hysterical women are profoundly out of touch with their conflicting emotions and so "express" them through the body in the form of physical symptoms.

The patriarchy is a bountiful source of ills for women, Northrup says. She describes how she herself began to "recover from patriarchal influences."

> When I first had a reading with Carolyn Myss [an internationally known "medical intuitive"] she told me that my body registered a rape between the ages of twenty-one and twenty-nine—the years that I was in medical school and doing my residency. Though I had not been physically raped, my body's energy system had been emotionally and psychologically "raped" by my medical training— something I had not been consciously aware of at the time.[10]

This is not what the Boston Women's Health Book Collective envisioned in 1973 when it produced its smart guide for women, the landmark *Our Bodies, Ourselves*. It is tempting to think that Northrup's touting of New Age silliness has little impact. But a coveted slot on PBS, generally regarded as an upscale, educational network, confers respectability on her outlandish theories. What's more, with over one-quarter of a million copies of her book in print, she has a huge audience.

A Specialty of One's Own

Northrup's "rape" during her male-dominated medical training is emblematic of the sexist oppression that, according to the women's health lobby, has spread its tentacles through every aspect of the medical system, from clinical research to treatment. According to the eight female physicians who established the Foundation for Women's Health in 1996: "Women are invisible in the health care system beyond their reproductive systems. The medical model using male science, male body, male culture is still the norm. Women die unnecessarily due to this male perspective."[11]

The foundation's goal is to create a specialty strictly for women's health that is similar in status to surgery or pediatrics. The American College of Women's Health Physicians supports this effort: "Those of us who were exposed to Women's Studies in college find Women's Health a very natural transition and progression," writes Kelley Phillips, president of the college. "There is little doubt that the increase in women's political and economic power during the past quarter century is a driving force in the development of a Women's Health Specialty."[12]

Some challenge the push for a new specialty. Dr. Michelle Harrison of the University of Pittsburgh School of Medicine is concerned that certifying physicians expressly to care for women would "allow the rest of those in medicine to feel absolved of responsibility for addressing the needs of women." Harrison predicts that creating a new specialty would "marginaliz[e] those practitioners who commit themselves to its practice."[13] Furthermore, says Dr. Florence Haseltine of the National Institutes of Health, "we have a women's health specialty, which is obstetrics and gynecology."

Haseltine, a former ob-gyn specialist herself, is eager to make needed changes in her field but believes that women's health "can be addressed by existing [medical] disciplines."[14] Indeed, for most doctors (except urologists and orthopedists), treating women patients is the norm, since women make greater use of health care services than men do. After all, women are overrepresented in the age groups that rely most heavily on medical services, constituting about 60 percent of the population sixty-five and over. Indeed, apart from the urological problems that beset old men, geriatrics could reasonably be said to be a woman's specialty because there are more than two women for every man over age eighty-five.

The Office of Women's Health at the Department of Health and Human Services has not yet called for a women's health specialty, but it is promoting a separate medical school curriculum in women's health. "Curricula in women's health should begin to erase the misconceptions caused by a generation of training physicians in the male model of disease," explains Elena V. Rios, a physician at the Office on Women's Health.[15] The call for a special curriculum, like the desire for a separate specialty, is rooted in the belief that women are second-class citizens in medicine and that doctors are concerned primarily with the "male model" of disease. This charge, as we shall see, is a fundamental misconception underlying much of the advocacy efforts in women's health today.

The Myth of the Second-Class Medical Citizen

In 1999 half a million people in ninety-eight cities ran the "Race for the Cure." Since the first running in Dallas in 1982, the race has become one of the largest series of 5K events in the nation. It is sponsored by the Susan G. Komen Foundation, and the proceeds go to community programs related to breast health education, screening and treatment and to breast cancer research. The race is a testament to women's passion about their health and their faith in the promise of medical research to one day overcome a dreaded disease.

These affirmations are a far cry from the sullen aggrievement voiced by many women's health advocates, who accuse the "androcentric" medical establishment of treating women as second-class citizens.[16] The former dean of the Berkeley School of Public Health, Patricia Buffler, has remarked on the fact that "there is so much outrage that half the human population has been left out" of clinical trials.[17] First Lady Hillary Rodham Clinton has remarked on the "appalling degree to which women were routinely excluded from major clinical trials of most illnesses."[18] During his presidential campaign Al Gore told an audience: "Throughout my career, I have fought for more research funds for those diseases so recently considered less important because they befell only women, such as breast cancer. . . . I pledge to you: women's health will always be at the top of my agenda."[19]

It is hard to imagine what more Gore could do. Women represented 62 percent of the more than six million participants in NIH-funded research in 1997, according to the NIH's Office of Research on Women's Health.[20] Breast cancer research has received more money than any other type of cancer research each year since 1985, when the National Cancer Institute began keeping track of disease-specific funding. It has always received many times the funding of prostate cancer—about five times the amount in 1997 and triple the expenditure in 1999.[21] These imbalances have prompted the Men's Health Network, a Washington-based group, to lobby Congress for redress.[22]

The incidence of invasive breast cancer in women is a little less than the incidence of invasive prostate cancer in men. In 1997, the last year for which the NIH has published data, 115 women in 100,000 received a diagnosis of invasive breast cancer, while 147 men in 100,000 received an invasive prostate cancer diagnosis.[23] Overall death rates are almost identical, but the mortality patterns differ with age. For example, almost twice as many men over sixty-five succumb to prostate cancer as do women to breast cancer. But breast cancer in young women is five times more lethal than prostate cancer in young men. Though relatively few women (and men) under sixty-five die from cancer of any kind, one could make an argument that breast cancer warrants more funding than prostate since its young victims fare less well.

Breast cancer also receives considerable funding compared to other diseases. A 1999 analysis in the *New England Journal of Medicine* conducted by Cary P. Gross of the Johns Hopkins University School of Medicine and his colleagues examined how the NIH sets priorities for funding specific diseases.[24] When the researchers calculated allocations according to the number of years of healthy life lost to a disease, breast cancer was found to be among the five conditions most "generously" funded; the other four were heart disease, dementia, AIDS and diabetes.

The enormous focus on breast cancer by women's health groups has probably contributed to women's skewed appreciation of health risks. Some middle-aged women believe they have a one-in-nine chance of dying from breast cancer at any point in time. One popular activist coalition on Long Island, New York, calls itself "One in Nine." But in fact, the one-in-nine figure applies to a woman's chance of developing breast cancer in her lifetime if she lives to age eighty-five. In other words, one in nine women who live to age eighty-five will have had cancer at some point. A forty-year-old woman with no special risk factors (like a mother or sister who had breast cancer at a young age), for example, has less than a one-in-two-hundred chance of getting breast cancer; the likelihood of dying from it is still smaller.

According to a 1997 survey of one thousand women by the National Council on the Aging, only one in four recognized that lung cancer is the leading cancer killer among women.[25] In 1997 about seventy thousand women died from lung cancer; less than forty-two thousand died from breast cancer. Though heart disease, not breast cancer or lung cancer, is the biggest killer of women—annual deaths from heart disease exceed deaths from all cancers combined—breast cancer concerns them more, according to the survey.

Elaine Ratner, author of *The Feisty Woman's Breast Cancer Book,* is worried that the "fear of breast cancer has reached epidemic proportions . . . because breast cancer has moved into the spotlight." Having been treated for cancer herself, Ratner says she feels lucky that it was in her breast. "No other body part is as expendable," she writes, but she suspects that many women forgo mammography because their inflated idea of breast cancer's lethality scares them away.[26] Less than 4 percent of women will die of breast cancer, while about one-third will die of heart disease.[27] "Haven't we induced an unrealistic fear in our efforts to raise awareness?" asks Jane Brody, the *New York Times* health writer. Heart disease, she writes, "does not conjure up anything like the fear that breast cancer does."[28]

Women's health has also received considerable attention in Congress. The Breast and Cervical Cancer Mortality Prevention Act of 1990 authorized the CDC to provide free Pap smears and screening mammograms for indigent women. In 1999, $158 million was appropriated for screening. In 1998 and 1999, dozens of women's health bills were introduced. The Breast Cancer Patient Protection Act, for example, would guarantee a minimum stay in the hospital of forty-eight hours for mastectomy and twenty-four hours for lymph node removal; the Breast Reconstruction Implemetation Act would guarantee insurance coverage for postmastectomy reconstructive surgery; the Women's Health and Cancer Rights Act ensures coverage for hospital care, procedures and second opinions.[29]

A few years ago the issue of mammograms for women in their forties became an urgent matter for lawmakers. In the winter of 1997 an NIH consensus development conference announced that women in their forties should decide for themselves, with the advice of their doctors, whether to get the breast X-ray.[30] Given the high rates of false-positive mammogram results, which lead some women to undergo needless surgery, and the negligible reduction in mortality associated with the screening of women in their forties, the panel concluded that a universal recommendation for annual or biannual mammography was unwarranted.

Many in Congress found the panel's pronouncement unacceptable. Within days of the conference Senator Olympia Snowe, a Maine Republican, introduced a nonbinding resolution in favor of mammography for women in their forties. The resolution, which passed 98–0, advised the National Cancer Institute (an NIH agency that played no oversight role in the conference's recommendation) to "direct the public to consider guidelines issued by other cancer organizations."[31] The resolution also called on the National Cancer Institute's (NCI) advisory board to issue its own recommendation in favor of regular mammograms for women in their forties.

Among those urging the advisory board were thirty-nine congresswomen. "We believe the only real option is to give guidance to the women of our country," they wrote in a letter to the board.[32] About a month later the NCI board did just as the congresswomen requested, earning the praise of HSS Secretary Donna Shalala: "Today years of confusion have been replaced by a clear, consistent scientific recommendation for women between the ages of 40 and 49."[33]

The irony of clamoring for explicit direction when women's health advocates had long been promoting self-determination was noted by Virginia L. Ernster, an epidemiologist at the University of California at San Francisco. "Will physicians who promote informed choice be open to legal suits?" she asks in her account of the mammogram debate, published in the *American Journal of Public Health*. The furor was unparalleled, she writes. "Probably never in the twenty-year history of such conferences has a resulting report ever generated more rancor and media attention."[34]

In Search of Sexism

In its 1999 report to Congress and the president, the U.S. Commission on Civil Rights expressed concern about "gender bias" in our health care system.[35] It pointed to unfairness in several spheres, including the career development of women physicians, women's participation as subjects in experimental trials and the quality of their clinical treatment.

Let us begin with career development. The commission claimed that medical schools practice the "steering of female [medical] students toward the more 'accepted' specialties such as pediatrics and general practice," while men are "more likely to enter the richly rewarding surgical subspecialties."[36] The commission presented no evidence that women are encouraged to select certain specialties. In fact, a fuller picture shows that many women doctors who want to plan a family are attracted to specialties with the shortest residencies (family practice, internal medicine, pediatrics and psychiatry).[37]

Surgical subspecialty training after medical school can take up to seven years at a time of life when women are in their prime childbearing years. True, the culture of surgery, with its brutal hours and strict hierarchy, may not appeal to many women, but those who burn to be surgeons will make it through. "If you want to do surgery," advises Mary Ann Hopkins, a New York surgeon, "do it!" What's more, she points out, women surgeons are highly sought after by both training programs and patients, especially those with breast disease.[38] Obstetrics and gynecology, the specialty with the highest malpractice insurance premiums in medicine, attracts 9 percent of women medical students and 3 percent of men.[39]

The Commission on Civil Rights leveled another charge of sexism against the funding of medical research conducted by women. Citing data from 1981 to 1992, the commission noted that women received 21.5 percent of all research project funding from NIH and that their grants were, on average, $30,000 lower than grants given to male scientists. Calling this an "uneven distribution" of funds and "a blatant civil rights violation," the commission said that HHS "must mandate that female scientists are awarded grants at the same ratio as men" to ensure that women conduct their fair share of the research.[40]

Remarkably, absent any evidence that quality proposals from women were being rejected at a greater rate than comparable proposals from men, the commission was not only claiming discrimination but advocating that grants be distributed according to the applicant's sex rather than the merit of the proposed research. Ironically, had the commission looked at data from 1992 to 1998, it would have seen that men and women enjoyed comparable success. For example, in 1993, the year for which the most complete data were collected, 18.3 percent of female applicants were awarded grants compared with 17.1 percent of the males; the sex of 3.5 percent of applicants was unrecorded (and about 15 percent of these applicants were successful).[41]

In other years the proportion of applicants who did not specify their sex was much higher, up to 27 percent in 1997, prompting the NIH's Office of the Director to warn that use of these data was questionable. "The unknown is so large that comparisons of male and female are not valid," I was told by the Office.[42] And the size of the grants? NIH has not tabulated such data since 1992, but according to Robert F. Moore of the Division of Statistical Analysis, the larger grants tend to go to more senior researchers, who are male. As female researchers move through the pipeline, Moore says, they too will be submitting grants with larger budgets.

But what are the prospects for such advancement? For decades women physicians entered academic medicine at higher rates than their male counterparts but were far less likely to be found at the associate and full professor levels, according to a study by Lynn Nonnemaker of the American Association of Medical Colleges.[43] Is discrimination to blame? No one can say without first examining the proportion of assistant professors who met criteria for advancement but were not promoted. The current imbalance in the promotion of men and women could be due to a host of factors, one of the most likely being lower production of publications by women who spend time away from the laboratory to tend to family responsibilities.

Nonnemaker's data support this interpretation. She found that women have a greater chance of being promoted from associate to full professor than from assistant to associate, suggesting that the point of departure from the tenure track occurs when women are in their late twenties and thirties—about the time when they are having babies and raising young children. It is important that we learn more about the reasons for women's slower advancement, but until then it would be folly to heed the injunction of Dr. Catherine DeAngelis, now the editor of the *Journal of the American Medical Association,* that women "must be promoted at a rate that is equitable to the rate for men."[44]

To our north, the same debate about glass ceilings has prompted the Canadian bureaucracy to act. Worried because there are fewer women researchers than men, the Natural Sciences and Engineering Research Council, Canada's main funding agency for research in biology, chemistry and physics, reinstated its practice of giving certain grants exclusively to women. In a letter to the commission, Doreen Kimura, a professor of psychology at Simon Fraser University in British Columbia, a grant recipient herself and president of Canada's Society for Academic Freedom and Scholarship, wrote: "I and many other scientists are deeply concerned at what amounts to flagrant discrimination in the distribution of a valuable research resource."[45]

The targets of the discrimination to which Kimura alludes are *men*. In fact, data show that women have been preferentially hired in Canadian universities, including in the sciences, since the early 1980s.[46] Kimura also questions the importance of same-sex role models, another of the commission's rationales for promoting women noncompetitively. More women would become scientists and physicians, goes the theory, if there were senior women to mentor them. Yet in Canada, as in the United States, women are entering medicine and the biological sciences in numbers that are equal to or even outstrip those for men. At the very least then, their predominantly male professors have not been holding them back.

Some might argue that women have made strides in spite of not having female role models and mentors. True, there are fewer women in engineering and physical sciences, but data suggest that this reflects preference—even the most mathematically gifted high school girls are less likely than similarly talented boys to choose to specialize in mathematics or the physical sciences in college or graduate school.[47] Indeed, neither Kimura nor I could find credible evidence that women learn better under female tutelage or that they are more interested in studying under female professors (save for women's studies students).

The Myth of Gender-Biased Research

The U.S. Commission on Civil Rights also cites as evidence of gender bias the allegation that women have been excluded from clinical trials.[48] It criticizes the "gender-incompetent manner" with which care is delivered, citing, for example, the failure to treat women aggressively for heart disease.[49] As we will see, these claims are highly misleading.

Among the many myths perpetuated by the women's health lobby is that women have been systematically excluded from participating in medical research. When she was head of the HHS Office of Women's Health in the mid-1990s, Dr. Susan J. Blumenthal routinely spread the word that women had been systematically underrepresented as subjects in medical research. This spurred a campaign on Capitol Hill to get women into research studies. "It was my female colleagues and I who led the charge to put an end to clinical trials conducted entirely on men—even for breast cancer," Senator Olympia Snowe says.[50]

But neither the senator's claims of success nor Blumenthal's accusations of systematic underrepresentation are correct. The fact is that neither the NIH nor drug companies conducted trials predominantly on men. Andrew G. Kadar, an anesthesiologist at UCLA School of Medicine, was one of the first to point out the sex-bias myth in medicine. "For a decade now charges of gender bias in medical care have gone unanswered," he wrote in the *Atlantic Monthly* in 1994. If anything, Kadar pointed out, studies that looked at only one sex more often focused on women than men.[51]

That is certainly the case with antidepressants. Back in the late 1950s and 1960s, when these medications were being tested in clinical trials, women were routinely included.[52] One of the largest and earliest studies I could find involved 215 subjects and was conducted in the late 1950s at the Massachusetts Mental Health Clinic.[53] Most of the participants in this placebo-controlled study of two antidepressants were women (or "housewives," as the authors called them). Nevertheless, women's health advocates routinely claim that the hormonal fluctuations brought on by women's menstrual cycles led researchers to bar them from clinical trials and thus early antidepressants were not studied in women.[54]

Governmental surveys in 1983 and 1988 found that "both sexes had substantial representation in clinical trials . . . in proportions that usually reflected the prevalence of the disease in the sex and age groups included in the trials."[55] In fact, conditions such as depression, osteoporosis and arthritis have always been more thoroughly studied in women, the FDA found. This should come as no surprise, since researchers tend to study the group most at risk. When the Institute of Medicine conducted its study on the status of women as research subjects, as requested by NIH in 1991, the institute's panel could not "nail down the truth of the perception that women have been under represented" in clinical trials.[56]

Still, as late as 1999 advocates like Phyllis Greenberger of the Society for Women's Health Research continued to make remarks like: "It's going to take some time before it's generally accepted that women and men have to be in clinical trials."[57] In the spring of 2000 I received a promotional letter from the *Harvard Women's Health Watch* newsletter telling readers that "nearly all drug testing has been done on men."[58] Wrong. The Office of Research on Women's Health at NIH, created in 1990 to respond to just these concerns, found that in 1994 research subjects for ongoing NIH clinical trials were 57 percent women, 36 percent men, and 6 percent unknown. The composition of subjects in trials funded in 1997 was 69 percent women and 31 percent men.[59]

Women's health advocates have a way of taking credit for conditions they did not create. For example, they attribute the recent numbers of women as subjects to a 1993 law requiring NIH-funded researchers to include women. It may well be true that women's *predominance* in trials is attributable to the law, but women's inclusion predated 1995, the year the law went into effect. According to the earliest NIH data I could find, since 1979 women have been very much a part of the research enterprise. That year 268 of the total 293 NIH-funded clinical trials contained female subjects. Thirteen of the 293 were all female, and 12 were all male.[60]

Since the mid-1990s major pharmaceutical companies like Lilly, Pfizer and Wyeth-Ayerst have boasted of their "women's health" divisions or initiatives. In doing so, they have largely repackaged research already under way. "More pharmaceutical companies are expected to develop women's health initiatives, if anything, to avoid mishaps in marketing," the *New York Times* reported. "Many of the new drugs promoted during the last several years—notably treatments for migraine and depression—are so similar in effectiveness [in men and women] that the manufacturers have to find other selling points."[61]

One can't fault these companies for seizing the opportunity to hit a public relations home run. After all, despite the prevailing assumption that women are underserved by the health care system, women buy more pharmaceuticals than men and visit doctors more often. The upside of aggressive advertising is that it may help inform women and better prepare them to ask questions of their doctors. But the fact is that clinical trials for drug development have routinely included women. For decades, drug companies have been developing medications for menopause, osteoporosis and other conditions that exclusively or disproportionately affect women.

When Exclusion Makes Sense

Have women ever been systematically omitted from clinical trials? Yes, starting in 1977, the Food and Drug Administration excluded pregnant and fertile women from participating in the toxicity testing of pharmaceuticals. The policy, withdrawn in 1993, evolved in the wake of the birth defect tragedies associated with thalidomide and diethylstilbestrol (DES). Women were excluded from the so-called phase I and II clinical trials—the small-scale safety-testing phases of pharmaceutical trials—to protect fetuses and, to some extent, avoid liability. Though the policy deserved its label of paternalistic, the point was to protect women and fetuses, not to favor men at their expense. Indeed, men themselves have not been rushing to volunteer for toxicity tests; why else would so many of the subjects who sign up be men from military bases and prisons?

When women have been omitted from other studies—the so-called late phase II and phase III studies of effectiveness—the reasons have been similarly practical and well intentioned. Sometimes women were not known to be at risk for a particular illness at the time the research was conducted. Such was the case with early clinical trials involving patients with AIDS. In the early 1980s homosexual men were the only group identified by the CDC as being at risk, but as it became clear that women could also be infected, researchers began to recruit them. In 1986, for example, only 2 percent of subjects in clinical trials were women; by 1992 more than 18 percent were women. Despite their 15 percent representation among all AIDS cases in 1998, they represented 36 percent of all subjects in NIH-funded AIDS clinical trials.[62]

Another reason for limiting certain trials to males is the fact that female subjects possessed clinical characteristics that made them difficult and expensive to study at a point in the investigation of a new treatment where the most basic questions of clinical value had yet to be answered.

The older age at which women suffer heart attacks explains their absence from a number of large NIH-funded cardiac trials conducted in the 1970s and early 1980s. Researchers had learned from the first major federally funded cardiac study, the Framingham Heart Study, that women's phase of risk for heart attack is ten to twenty years later than that for men. When Framingham researchers recruited their first cohort of subjects in 1948, fully 55 percent were women. Because the women were relatively young (ages thirty to sixty-two) when the study began, follow-up in the early years of the study revealed few myocardial infarctions among the women.

Age has had a major effect on participation in studies of coronary risk factors. Older subjects, whether men or women, are underrepresented in heart disease trials. Indeed, the Lipid Research Clinics Coronary Primary Prevention Trial (designed in the early 1960s to look at the benefit of cholesterol-lowering drugs in people under sixty-five with a prior history of heart attack) and the large Multiple Risk Factor Intervention Trial and Lipid Research Clinics in the 1970s (both of which examined risk factors for heart attack) left women out because the focus was on preventing heart attack in middle age—and few middle-aged women suffer heart attacks.

Also, the elderly subjects are sometimes too frail to tolerate the study procedure itself; this was the case with treatment trials related to angina (cardiac-related chest pain), which usually require vigorous treadmill exercise tests.[63] A 1992 article in the *Journal of the American Medical Association* by J. H. Gurwitz and his colleagues, "The Exclusion of the Elderly and Women from Clinical Trials in Acute Myocardial Infarction," captured the phenomenon nicely.[64] In reviewing trials from 1960 to 1991, the authors found that more than 60 percent of them excluded people—women and men—older than seventy-five.

Gurwitz's research team concluded that age, not sex, determined who was enrolled. This simply reflected the way research is done: when scientists begin studying a condition, they choose subjects who are most at risk and least medically complicated in order to control as many variables as possible. Because women are older when they manifest heart disease, they are more likely to be suffering from additional age-related illnesses and taking several medications, clinical realties that make it difficult to assess the impact of the interventions being studied. This explains why older male subjects were also omitted. Research on blood pressure reflects this practice as well. The large 1973 Hypertension Detection and Follow-up Study financed by NIH enrolled comparable numbers of men and women because both sexes enter the phase of risk at about the same age.

Finally, expense plays a role. The 1981 Physicians Health Study—the study in which aspirin was found to reduce the risk of heart attack—included only male physicians as subjects. Physicians were selected as the study population because they were assumed to be likely to have a high rate of compliance with the self-administered protocol.[65] Male physicians in particular were selected because very few female doctors (about one for every ten males) were old enough to be at risk for heart disease when the trial began. Young female doctors could have been included only if many more subjects were enrolled (to enhance the chances of "catching" the few at risk) or female enrollees were observed for a longer period than male enrollees.

Consider this fact too: about 260,000 *male* physicians were screened for the 1981 study in order to recruit the 22,000 who actually participated. Had the study been performed on women, the number of subjects screened and then randomized to the placebo and active arms of the trial would have had to be three times as large—and the study at least three times as expensive—to obtain the same magnitude of results found in the men.[66] For the past two decades women have been represented in most cardiac studies to the degree that they are at risk, but the practical reasons for their earlier omission are unappreciated by the Commission on Civil Rights and many women's health activists.

So are explanations for physicians' tendency to put women through fewer complex diagnostic procedures such as arterial catheterization. The combination of age and concurrent disease has traditionally put them at higher risk for adverse side effects. Women's smaller anatomy is another consideration. The arteries around the heart, for example, are sometimes too narrow to accommodate the clog-clearing devices. In fact, the rate of complications, including death, from trying to unclog arteries (through procedures such as balloon angioplasty), though small overall, is still considerably higher in women.[67] In the exception that proves the rule about size, one of the very first artificial heart operations, in 1966, was performed on a thirty-seven-year-old woman whose chest cavity was big enough. "We're always trying to perfect the miniaturization process," says Michael E. DeBakey, the pioneering surgeon who did the operation.[68]

Indeed, cardiac surgeons are developing "keyhole heart surgery," a minimally invasive form of surgery used to repair heart valves, perform coronary artery bypass and repair congenital malformations. The major advantages over traditional open-chest methods are reductions in blood loss and in the chance of wound infection, because there is less tissue trauma. Also, the typical hospital stay is less than a week. Stephen B. Colvin, chief of cardiothoracic surgery at New York University Medical Center, is perfecting this technique. He predicts that older and more fragile patients with cardiac disease—that is, women—will be especially good candidates. In fact, Colvin and his team chose to offer the keyhole surgical technique (which now almost one thousand patients have received) not to younger and healthier patients but to those with diabetes, osteoporosis and previous open-heart surgery. The procedure, he said, "is especially beneficial for older, frailer patients for whom open-chest surgery would be devastating or contraindicated."[69]

Another difference in the use of procedures between men and women reflects the difficulty of making a diagnosis of heart attack in women. The reasons are multiple. The location and nature of chest pain do not always follow easily recognizable patterns, and exercise treadmill tests and imaging studies may be difficult to interpret. Even if her chest pain follows the more typical pattern, a sixty-year-old woman has an approximately fifty-fifty chance of having significant coronary artery blockage; a sixty-year-old man with the same symptoms has a 90 percent chance of having blockage.[70] If a woman doesn't realize she is having a heart attack or the physician is confused by her symptoms, she will miss the time-sensitive window (within about twelve hours of onset of symptoms) for receiving clot-dissolving treatment (thrombolysis).[71] If this treatment is not administered within several hours of the onset of chest pain, the benefit of dissolving the clot may no longer exceed the risk of causing bleeding elsewhere in the body.[72]

On the other hand, if her chest pain symptoms are not really cardiac in origin, a woman may undergo needless intervention. Indeed, actual coronary artery obstruction is minimal or absent two to three times as often in women as in men, a discovery that repeatedly emerged when women were catheterized on the presumption that they were at risk for heart attack.[73] (Notably, when a definite diagnosis of heart attack is made, women are as likely as men to undergo catheterization, clot-dissolving therapy and bypass.) By comparison, with medical conditions diagnosed more readily than heart attack, like infection, sex-related differences are not an issue. For example, women and men with pneumonia and other infections receive the same care—antibiotic treatment is started rapidly in both, and treatment is of similar duration.[74]

Outrageous Practices?

Advocates condemn the omission of women from some studies and the lesser likelihood that they will undergo certain procedures as evidence of the devaluation of women's health, yet they turn around and charge sexism again when women get too much attention from other quarters of the medical profession. Efforts by Pfizer, the manufacturer of Viagra, to apply that medication to women were condemned by feminists as attempts to "medicalize" female sexuality—that is, as turning sexual responsiveness, or the lack of it, into a disease that needs to be cured.

In protest, a number of women's groups gathered at an international meeting on female sexual dysfunction held at the Boston University School of Medicine in the fall of 1999. According to the *Boston Globe*, the women considered using a six-foot papier-mâché vulva as part of a protest display. Though they ultimately rejected that idea, they remained vocal about their concerns. For example, Paula Caplan, a psychologist at Brown University, fretted to the *Globe* reporter that a sexual enhancer (such as Viagra) for women "is going to put enormous pressure on women who may not want to have sex."[75]

Gynecologists have also been criticized for paying too much attention to women. "The Lord giveth and the gynecologist taketh away," claims the antihysterectomy group HERS (Hysterectomy Educational Resources and Services Foundation), implying that women's surgery is propelled by mercenary interest. "Gynecologists, hospitals and drug companies make more than 5 billion dollars a year from the business of hysterectomy and castration."[76]

But what about the benefits women derive from hysterectomy? Interviews with women just before and then several years after hysterectomy have found that urinary incontinence improves, sexual interest increases and pain with intercourse diminishes after hysterectomy.[77] In 1999 University of Maryland epidemiologists reported in *JAMA* that women enjoy enhanced sexual functioning after hysterectomy.[78] More than eleven hundred women were interviewed before the procedure and then several times within a two-year period after it. Whereas 19 percent complained of pain with intercourse before, only 4 percent had this symptom two years later. There are several reasons for less pain with sexual intercourse after hysterectomy, including the changes in anatomy that accompany the procedure and its ameliorating effect on chronic pain and bleeding (most commonly from endometriosis).

The treatment of breast cancer with radical mastectomy, the standard procedure until the early to mid-1980s, still rankles some women's health advocates. In her 1999 book *A Darker Ribbon,* Ellen Leopold, a writer and member of the Women's Community Cancer Project in Cambridge, Massachusetts, opines:

> The surgical removal of the breast has to be seen as a violent act. The apparent barbarity of the procedure raises the question of male intent. It is not much of a stretch to view surgery as yet another opportunity to punish a woman for the ambivalent feelings she provokes. . . . The aura surrounding breast surgery reinforced the worst gender stereotypes, attributing all power to the male hero.[79]

Today we know that radical mastectomy is not necessary for most women, but before the late 1970s and early 1980s it was the accepted life-saving procedure. A surgeon who did not perform it would have been considered derelict. In hindsight, we can see that many women underwent needlessly aggressive surgery, but there wasn't a gender bias: men too have been subject to the radical nature of cancer surgery. Thousands of men with positive blood tests as their only sign of possible prostate cancer have undergone needless radical prostatectomies, sometimes involving the removal of pelvic nerves and thus destroying their ability to perform sexually. Then, if metastases appeared, men were castrated, since testosterone seemed to promote cancer growth. The development of more conservative and safer procedures and operations for both women and men is a continuing priority for physicians, but surgical practice must not be taken out of its historical context.

Until the 1960s and 1970s that context reflected a different conceptualization of cancer pathology than doctors hold today. "The flawed concept . . . that cancer was a local process and best approached by extensive excision of surrounding tissue was applied to all types of tumors," Jerome Groopman, an oncologist and professor of medicine at Harvard, points out. In response to Leopold's feminist interpretation of breast cancer, Groopman cannot help but wonder, in his review of her book: "Does this mean that urological surgeons were, consciously or subconsciously, acting out as alpha males to dominate and abase the vulnerable men of the tribe?"[80]

In the 1994 book *Outrageous Practices: How Gender Bias Threatens Women's Health,* the journalists Leslie Laurence and Beth Weinhouse note that electroconvulsive therapy is given to women disproportionately and say that "what is worrisome is that more women than men are getting a potentially damaging treatment."[81] Women do, in fact, receive ECT more often than men do. And with good reason: more women than men are diagnosed with depression. Furthermore, there are more elderly females with depression because women live longer. ECT is often safer than medication in the frail elderly; properly conducted, it rarely leads to complications and is generally very effective. Yet when the authors were guests on *Oprah,* the host whipped the audience into hooting indignation at the plight of female patients, exclaiming, "Are you angry yet?"[82]

Vive la Différence?: Not So Fast

The women's health lobby also contends that researchers have ignored "gender-specific medicine," or differences in the way men and women respond to medications. To be sure, some meaningful sex differences do exist. The hormonal fluctuations of the menstrual cycle, pregnancy and menopause and the use of oral contraceptives may interfere with the effectiveness of some medications and not others. But touting the discovery of gender-based differences in pharmacology as a research revolution is premature; its practical impact on disease is only starting to be evaluated.

Much of the emphasis on "gender-based medicine" seems to overlook the fact that when physicians administer medications they tailor the dose to the particular patient they are treating. They account for body mass, fat, kidney and liver function and additional medications the patient is taking. In some cases—as when medicating psychosis or pain—dosage is based on intensity of symptoms and then raised if they persist or lowered if side effects are too uncomfortable. In short, patients generally end up on individualized, empirical dosing schedules that do not rely on a set formula derived from gender comparison research.

Nevertheless, if sex-based differences are sometimes important, it is striking that a failure to look for them is reliably depicted as hurting only women. "Women are not merely little men," said Phyllis Greenberger of the Society for Women's Health Research in asserting that women get the short end of the research stick when researchers assume that results of mixed-sex clinical trials automatically apply to women.[83] Perhaps distinctions in drug responses have been glossed over too readily, but if so, then large men have been disadvantaged as well. After all, averaging the results obscures discrete sex-related differences for *both* sexes.

As if following Greenberger's lead, the *New York Times* ran the following headline on a number of reports on women's health research: "Research Neglects Women's Health, Studies Find: Reports Say Health Trials Often Disregard Differences in the Sexes."[84] An editorial in *USA Today* echoed the sentiment: "Government-Funded Studies Deny Women Key Health Data." It went on to rehash the myths about women's health: "The habit of overlooking women in medical research is deeply ingrained and hard to shake. For decades, women have been alternatively ignored or overprotected. And the research hierarchy is still largely dominated by the interests and concerns of white males."[85]

The focus of both the *New York Times* and *USA Today* articles was a report on the status of women as research subjects released in the spring of 2000 by the General Accounting Office (GAO). The report claims that many clinical trials have not included women in "numbers large enough to allow analysis that would definitively measure different outcomes for women and men."[86] The GAO is referring to a provision of the 1993 NIH Revitalization Act that requires NIH-funded researchers to conduct a "valid analysis" of sex differences, a provision pushed through largely at the behest of the Congressional Women's Caucus.[87] That NIH-funded researchers failed to consistently conduct sex-response analyses, the GAO says, suggests that the NIH was remiss in enforcing the analysis requirement of the 1993 law.

But the NIH is keenly aware of the analysis mandate. From the very beginning, the exact meaning of the term "valid analysis" has been a topic of heated debate among researchers. If "valid analysis" means the ability to discern a *statistically* meaningful difference in response between sexes, researchers point out nervously, then the difficulty of doing clinical trials greatly increases. It also poses ethical challenges.

Imagine that a treatment for lung cancer is being tested in a group of men and women, and early results show that it is very effective in causing tumors to shrink. Commonly, if studies show a strong effect, either beneficial or harmful, in the cohort of patients enrolled early on, researchers are ethically required to halt the study. If the drug is a boon, then its use in other patients is rapidly promoted; if it is harmful, word goes out to researchers and doctors and patients to consider stopping its use.[88] Analyzing data by sex introduces a big ethical wrinkle: If dramatically positive results are found, what patient is going to want to continue on placebo just so researchers can study enough subjects for a subgroup analysis? Moreover, is it ethical to give a female patient a placebo when the experimental drug has already shown itself to be superior to placebo in both men and women?

Ethics aside, sex comparisons would inflate the costs of research because statistical analysis requires large numbers of male and female subjects for each clinical trial. Consider that every study has a minimum of two groups right from the start: the group that receives the medication or intervention, and the control (or placebo) group. Adding other comparison groups—men versus women, to see whether the medication has different outcomes in each—requires a three- to fourfold increase in the total number of subjects. If the threshold number of subjects in all four groups (experimental versus placebo, and women versus men) is not met, a reliable statistical analysis simply cannot be done. If there are too few subjects in each group, a difference is likely to go undetected unless it is hugely obvious.

To make matters more complicated, few medications have dramatically different effects in men and women anyway. The Food and Drug Administration did not seem especially concerned about the issue of subgroup analysis when it was raised in 1987. "The number of documented gender-related pharmacological differences of clinical consequence is at this time small and conducting formal effectiveness studies to detect them may be difficult. . . . Such studies are therefore not routinely necessary."[89] And therein lies the real issue: How can we justify the cost of routinely searching for differences that are unlikely to matter?

After all, including more subjects makes for larger, more expensive studies that take longer to complete. The NIH would end up funding fewer total studies and would thus generate less biomedical knowledge. The biggest risk is that potentially lifesaving therapies will go untested because money is being wasted examining unimportant relative differences in response to treatment. Back in 1993 the NIH recognized these implications of the legislative provision, and the next year it officially defined "valid subgroup analysis" to mean an unbiased evaluation that could have "clinical" or "public health significance" rather than statistical significance.[90] In other words, it dropped the standard scientific practice of discounting group differences that arise by chance. Thus, the NIH is now being blamed for failing to enforce a law that was ill considered in the first place and whose requirements were defined (and made available for public comment in the *Federal Register*) by the institute itself.

Fortunately, not every study has to be analyzed by sex: researchers need a reason to anticipate that men and women will respond differently. Typically, such information would come from the smaller safety and efficacy trials that precede a large clinical trial. According to Paul Leber, a psychopharmacologist and former division head at the FDA, "Almost any disinterested clinical trials analyst worth his or her salt would routinely examine the data to determine to what extent membership in various groups (for example, sex, age, race) contributed to the positive finding."[91]

Moreover, researchers can obtain more precise information about women's (and men's) responses to medications through single-sex trials. If the preliminary safety and efficacy data or the clinical trial itself suggests a sex difference, researchers should follow up with separate trials for men and women. In fact, that seems to be the direction the NIH has already taken. For example, of the forty-nine trials initiated in 1987 by the National Heart, Lung and Blood Institute at NIH and reported in May 1993, seven involved only women, and one involved only men.[92] In 1997 the NIH had almost one thousand single-sex clinical studies in progress. Of those, over *70 percent* were women-only.[93]

It is not clear how Congress and the NIH will resolve the matter of "valid subgroup analysis." Days after the GAO report came out, Senators Tom Harkin (D-IA), Barbara Mikulski (D-MD) and Olympia Snowe (R-ME) and Representative Henry Waxman (D-CA) called for hearings.[94] "Women continue to be shortchanged by federal research efforts," said Snowe.[95] Nonetheless, the story as it has unfolded so far is a classic example of the unerring tendency of so many women's health advocates to view events through a lens of aggrievement and to ignore the numerous adverse consequences of elevating politics over science in setting research policy.

There Is No Women's Health Crisis

In 1996 Secretary of Health and Human Services Donna Shalala said, "We are rapidly approaching the day when women's health research is not only sitting in the front of the bus—but is heading toward a clinic or hospital administered equally by men and women."[96] When the secretary made that statement, women's health research was already sitting in front and women were well represented in the ranks of hospital administrators at the level of vice president.[97] Today women have considerable influence in the medical marketplace. Women's health centers are springing up; in 1999 at least thirty-six hundred programs across the country called themselves women's health centers.[98] There are few comparable centers for men.

To say that mainstream medicine itself caters to men cannot be the case since even after their childbearing years women visit the doctor more than men.[99] Pharmaceutical companies are advertising vigorously to women, thereby increasing the likelihood of an informed consumer and along the way generating competition between companies that can benefit the consumer by lowering costs and expanding variety. In some specialties women are in special demand.[100] And at the end of the century 44 percent of the entering class in our medical schools was female.[101]

But some will always portray women as deprived. After all, the women's health lobby and its fund-raising apparatus run on the perception that women have been slighted in order to benefit men.[102] The Society for Women's Health Research, for example, decries the fact that "52 percent of the population receives barely 14 percent of federal health research funding."[103] Except for the tiny Office of Research on Women's Health, "the whole rest of the NIH is the men's office," claims Marianne Legato, a physician who directs the Partnership for Women's Health at the Columbia School of Physicians and Surgeons.[104]

Apparently, these advocates count only the portion of the NIH budget earmarked for diseases of women as beneficial to females—not the great mass of research on human health generally. By that barometer, less than 7 percent of funding goes to clinical research on all male diseases. That means at least 93 percent goes to diseases that affect either women or both sexes. Thus, 52 percent of the population (women) benefits from at least 93 percent of the research budget. Pitting the well-being of women against men is not only petty but, considering that women outlive men by six years, rather absurd.

The half-truths disseminated by the women's health movement and the righteous indignation it seeks to provoke are not without harmful consequences for women. Facts taken out of context (such as women's lower rate of catheterization) can lead patients to clamor for, and ultimately receive, procedures that may cause them more harm than good. After all, if you were a woman, wouldn't you press the doctor for a test if you were led to believe he was withholding it? This mentality often contaminates the doctor-patient relationship. "When I give lectures on the doctor-patient relationship to physicians, many of the overworked doctors—male and female—typically comment on how frustrating it is to deal with women who come into their office with an attitude of 'Prove that you're not going to take advantage of me,'" says Edward Bartlett, associate adjunct professor at the George Washington University School of Public Health.[105]

Assuredly, there is more to know about the treatment of diseases in women. We need to know more, for example, about the way natural hormones, contraceptives and replacement hormones affect other medications women take. Increasingly, there is evidence that pre- and postmenopausal women may metabolize drugs differently. We need to know more about efficient diagnosis of heart attack and chest pain in women and to develop better ways to interpret diagnostic tests for chest pain. But it is wrongheaded to confuse the need to know more—an imperative that will always be with us—with the notion that women are second-class subjects of medical research.

5

Crack Moms of South Carolina

WHEN THE CRACK COCAINE EPIDEMIC hit Charleston, South Carolina, in the late 1980s, doctors and nurses at the Medical University of South Carolina were begging pregnant addicts to get drug treatment. They were sadly familiar with the drastic effects of potent stimulants like cocaine during the third trimester: uterine hemorrhage, oxygen-deprived babies, spontaneous abortion and extreme prematurity. Between October 1988 and September 1989, 119 pregnant women who came to the Medical University's emergency room were identified as using cocaine. Ten miscarried, and the remaining 109 were still using cocaine at the time of delivery. Not one went to drug treatment either before or after her baby was born.[1]

In the spring of 1989 a small group of frustrated nurses and doctors met with Charleston's police chief, Reuben Greenberg, and the county solicitor, Charles M. Condon, who would later become state attorney general. That October they unveiled a policy that aimed to use the force of law to ensure that pregnant women got treatment: a woman could be arrested and charged with child neglect or delivery of drugs to a minor if she was using drugs just prior to delivery, tested positive for drugs more than once during the third trimester or tested positive during the third trimester and subsequently refused or missed an appointment with the substance abuse or prenatal clinic. Condon appeared in stern public service announcements on TV. "Not only will you live with guilt, you could be arrested," he warned. "This is a tragedy you can prevent. . . . If you stay with the [treatment] program, you won't be arrested. Wake up from the nightmare. Think about your baby first."[2]

The get-tough policy soon showed signs of success. The incidence of cocaine-positive urine screens among pregnant women coming to the emergency room dropped dramatically after the restrictive policy was implemented, from more than twenty per month to five or six, according to a report in the *Journal of the South Carolina Medical Association*. Deliveries at the institution did not decline following implementation of the policy.[3]

The Medical University's drug testing policy drew fire. The Center for Reproductive Law and Policy in New York City condemned the South Carolina program as an excuse to "punish women for their behavior during pregnancy."[4] Catherine Christophillis, a state prosecutor who helped craft and enforce the child protection effort, was personally targeted. "The ACLU, women's rights activists and local defense attorneys came after me. I was a terrorist, a Nazi, the pregnancy police. They said babies would be born dead in the streets of South Carolina because women would be too afraid to go the hospital."[5] Shirley Brown, the obstetrical nurse who helped organize the meeting with Greenberg and Condon, received death threats.[6]

Advocates for the pregnant addicts assailed the Charleston plan. While I too saw no need to arrest and incarcerate women, the imposition of drug testing and treatment requirements, as we will see, is often critical. Yet the advocates insisted that addicts didn't need to be coerced into treatment with threats. "The true crisis" is lack of treatment, according to Lynn M. Paltrow of the Center for Reproductive Law and Policy.[7] If there were only more treatment programs available, she said, the problem would be solved: drug-addicted pregnant women would flock to them.

Paltrow was half right: as continues to be true in most places, Charleston did not have enough programs (residential programs specifically) for pregnant women and women with young children. But she and her activist colleagues are dead wrong about the need for leverage if many addicts are to benefit from treatment. The substance abuse treatment system has long recognized the virtues of coercion. "Legal referral to treatment is a consistent predictor of success," says George De Leon of the National Drug Research Institute in New York City and a world-renowned expert in drug treatment.[8]

The Medical University of South Carolina was following a useful tradition of applying leverage to change destructive behavior. But the war waged against the Medical University, first by women's rights and civil liberties advocates and then by the federal government, is the story of how a campaign for victim rights competed with the hospital's clinical imperative to treat addicted mothers-to-be, defend the health of the near-term fetus and protect the mother-newborn relationship.

Addicts as Victims?

In 1993 the Center for Reproductive Law and Policy filed a $3 million class action suit against the city of Charleston on behalf of ten women who were drug-tested.[9] The defendants included the Medical University, some nurses and doctors and the solicitor's office. The allegations included violation of the women's privacy and reproductive rights and (because eight of the women tested were black) racial discrimination. By 1994 the Office of Civil Rights in the Department of Health and Human Services had entered the picture. It threatened to withhold the Medical University's federal funding, a total of 60 percent of its budget, unless it abandoned its policy. Warning that the program violated Title VI of the Civil Rights Act (the law prohibiting discrimination in federally funded institutions), the Office of Civil Rights told the hospital that "it is the government's obligation to ensure that Federal funds do not support a program which discriminates."[10] In the words of Dorothy E. Roberts of Rutgers School of Law at Newark, the "choice of a punitive response perpetuates the historical devaluation of Black women as mothers."[11]

Chief Greenberg, who is black, found the charges of devaluation and discrimination ludicrous. "Punishment? Discrimination? I'd consider it discriminatory if they *didn't* go out of their way to save these black babies," he told me when I visited Charleston. "The doctors and nurses wanted to level the playing field for these unborn babies, at least during the last three months before they were born," he continued. "They wanted to give them the same chances as a kid with middle-class white parents."[12]

From a logistical standpoint it is no surprise that most of the women were poor and black. The Medical University was the only local institution that offered obstetrical care to the predominantly black indigent population, the population in which crack use happened to be concentrated. Judge C. Weston Houck of the U.S. District Court in South Carolina ruled in 1997 that there was no basis for the accusation of racial discrimination. "The evidence presented by the defendants shows that whenever a patient presented with one of the criteria [for testing], they were tested. There is no evidence that the criteria were applied subjectively," Houck wrote. He also noted that a "substantial majority of the plaintiffs stopped abusing cocaine," perhaps as a consequence of the very policy they were challenging in court.[13]

But Houck's ruling came too late. In 1994 hospital administrators felt that they had no choice but to close the program. After the Medical University suspended its drug-testing-with-consequences policy, the state child protection agency was still brought in on cases of potential child endangerment, but police were not notified if the mother was uncooperative.

A toothless policy was just fine with Professor Mary Faith Marshall, director of the Program in Bioethics at the Medical University, who had objected to the program all along. Testifying in 1998 at a U.S. House of Representatives hearing on substance abuse and pregnancy, she dismissed the assumption that a woman who uses crack is unfit to be a mother, and anyway, she said, restrictions on pregnant women constitute sex discrimination. "The symbol of the anti-mother is easily exploited by political opportunists who trade on myth, symbol and fear to further their political agenda," she declared. Marshall also condemned society's "moral judgmentalism about substance abuse."[14]

Even some physicians talk about addiction using the vocabulary of victimhood. Stephen R. Kandall, chief of neonatology at Beth Israel Medical Center in New York, pronounces drug abuse to be the "result of manipulation by the media, inappropriate over-medication by physicians, or [addicts'] own attempts to cope with social barriers to achieving equality and self-fulfillment." He adds, "Although women with economic and family support can mask their addiction, however tragic their circumstances, substance-abusing women are united in a punishing sisterhood whose human costs are inestimable."[15]

In their 1994 documentary film *Women of Substance: The Struggles and Triumphs of Women Addicts Seeking Treatment,* Rory Kennedy and Robin Smith portray women in a residential treatment program. We watch long segments of the women sitting in group therapy, talking about their feelings and hugging and crying. I assume these women were required to hold jobs or complete GEDs—that's what most good programs expect—but the message that *Women of Substance* conveys is unmistakable: these women are victims of a disease. "They take drugs to medicate themselves," Barry Zuckerman, chairman of pediatrics at Boston City Hospital, says in the film. "I don't think it is any different than me taking a beer" after a hard day.

The film also cast a disapproving look at the South Carolina situation. "We can no longer afford to be angry and punitive," says the narrator, the actress Joanne Woodward. "There are too many lives at stake." The false-choice rhetoric—"treatment, yes, punishment, no"—is the mantra of advocates who refuse to acknowledge that serious addiction frequently requires the application of coercion if the patient is to get better.

Francine Feinberg is the executive director of Meta House, a residential treatment program in Milwaukee. In 1998 she told a subcommittee of the House Governmental Affairs and Oversight Committee: "Punitive measures ignore the root causes of addiction for so many women—sexual abuse and battering—during which women are victimized. Punitive approaches such as these make these women victims again."[16] Lynn M. Paltrow of the Center for Reproductive Law and Policy told Ted Koppel on ABC's *Nightline,* "Everybody's ready to call these women selfish, when the real problem is that they are not selfish enough." Though they expose their unborn children to potentially dangerous substances, Paltrow reasons, the ones harmed "first and foremost [are] themselves."[17]

The feminists' preoccupation with the mother at the expense of the near-term child is not new. Julia Smith Andre was a woman with a metabolic disorder known as phenylketonuria. She was aware that she needed to be on a restrictive diet during pregnancy to avoid subjecting her fetus to a high probability of mental retardation. She refused to follow dietary restrictions and, as her doctors expected, gave birth to a profoundly retarded child. Here is how the bioethicist Mary Briody Mahowald of the University of Chicago rationalizes Andre's actions using "feminist standpoint theory":

> Patients generally belong to the non-dominant group to whom privilege status may be imputed because the recommendations that cover their care are governed by the dominant group. . . . Granting privileged status to [Andre's] decision regarding diet control and medical interventions during pregnancy is supported by feminist standpoint theory. . . . So long as the impact of her decision does not disproportionately burden others, an egalitarian view of feminism further supports her decision.[18]

The Andre case is full of legal land mines, to be sure. But in condoning her behavior on *ethical* grounds, Mahowald joins the ranks of Marshall, Paltrow and the feminist-legal establishment, all of whom put the rights of the autonomous mother—autonomous in that she has the power to determine the health of her newborn—above those of the near-term fetus, who is utterly helpless. "Clearly the standpoint of the person most affected is crucial to this assessment," Mahowald asserts, referring to Andre, not her brain-damaged child, as the "person most affected."[19]

Harm Reduction or Harm Production?

Another advocacy group assailing the Medical University of South Carolina was the Lindesmith Center in New York City. Lindesmith has long been a proponent of "harm reduction," the philosophy that drug abuse is inevitable and that society should therefore try to minimize the damage that addicts do to themselves. As defined by the Harm Reduction Coalition, which is based in Oakland, California, harm reduction "meets users where they are at . . . accepting, for better or worse, that drug use is part of our world."[20]

This acceptance of drug use has reached its zenith in the Netherlands, where addicts have formed a union called the Federation of Dutch Junkie Leagues, which lobbies the government for services such as housing, health benefits and welfare payments. Addict activists and their supporters say that drug abuse is a human right and the government has a responsibility to make it safer to be an addict.

In the United States needle exchange programs are the most familiar example of harm reduction. The programs may make some impact when they help enroll addicts in treatment programs and, in the interim, require that addicts bring back used needles and exchange them for the same number of clean ones. However, in many cities addicts are simply given handfuls of clean needles, at no cost and with no expectation that they will quit using or enter drug treatment. In 1998 Baltimore's commissioner of health proposed going a step further and administering heroin, at taxpayer expense, to addicts. He was inspired by government-run programs in Australia, Switzerland and the Netherlands, which do just that. Whether public funds should support these efforts is another debate, but the idea that addicts represent a class of oppressed citizens is particularly ironic. After all, it is generally their own failure to control their drug use—resulting in addiction, accidents, arrest, job loss and so on—that leads to their "oppression."

That the consequences of drug addiction are to be accommodated by a "nonjudgmental" society becomes chilling when children are involved. "Mother Dog," the nom de plume of a drug-abusing mother, has a regular column in the *Harm Reduction Coalition Communication*. She describes her column as a forum on "parenting" and previews such topics as "what to tell your child when they ask about your lifestyle ('Mommy, how come all your friends come over at 3:00 A.M.?'), money management issues for parents who use drugs, and how to deal with a child that is using [drugs] or has begun to ask questions" about them.

Mother Dog continues:

> As a single mother of two, parenting is a subject of great impor-
> tance to me. . . . My drug of choice for the last 15 years has been
> speed by injection. . . . [We live] in abject poverty. There are very
> few resources available to me as a mother in my situation and
> particularly as a mother who uses drugs—other than the many drug
> dealers in the neighborhood [who] anonymously deliver clothing,
> food and medical supplies to my doorstep. I decided to start this
> column so that other parents in similar situations can come
> together and share ideas and information, discuss triumphs and
> challenges and empower one another in our parenting and in our
> lives.

Later Mother Dog laments that she has "few if any positive role models"
and that she suffers from "stigmatization and negative labeling."[21]

To be fair, most critics of the South Carolina policy do not regard the
use of crack and heroin as an acceptable alternative lifestyle, but at bottom
they share a philosophical kinship with Mother Dog. They see the drug-
using mother as the victim and the child as a bit player in the drama, one
whose interests may be sacrificed to the mother's autonomy. They want to
spare the mother the burden of proving that she is a fit parent. And if she
turns out to be incompetent, they reason, it is the responsibility of social
service agencies to catch her failing at it.

How Bad Is Crack for Babies?

Critics of the Medical University of South Carolina are quick to remind us
that crack's effect on children is not as dire as once feared. Follow-up studies
of "crack babies" have indeed failed to identify the horribly brain-damaged
cohort of ghetto children predicted in the 1980s. Furthermore, studies
that did find developmental problems neglected to control for the
mothers' use of other substances during pregnancy—especially alcohol—
and for lack of prenatal care, untreated venereal disease and poor nour-
ishment.[22] To be sure, crack use could have created or exacerbated the
violence, alcohol consumption, disruption and disease in the women's

lives, but it is almost impossible to disentangle the prenatal effects of co-caine from that of all the other factors that can compromise babies in the womb and doom them to a stunted infancy and troubled childhood.

In the mid-1990s better studies began to appear. They documented that while prenatal crack exposure per se did not lead to severe mental deficits and uncontrollable behavior, as originally feared, cocaine did have a discernible, if subtle, effect on the central nervous system in many chil-dren. A comprehensive analysis of the data was conducted by Barry Lester, a Brown University psychologist, and his colleagues. They reviewed 101 published studies that used objective measures of behavior and cognition and employed a control group to account for the numerous additional risk factors common to cocaine-using mothers. Most of the studies were conducted with infants and preschoolers. The eight studies conducted on school-age children revealed deficits in IQ and language.[23]

Children whose mothers used cocaine had IQs measuring about three points lower than those of the control children. This is not a big nu-merical difference, but it takes on new meaning when placed in context. For children growing up in poverty, the average IQ is ten to fifteen points or more below the norm of 100 without drugs. "For these children," Lester says, "three points can make the difference between normal and abnormal [because] even small differences that do not start out as abnormalities could become abnormalities if exaggerated by environmental factors."[24]

In an article in *Science,* the authors extrapolate from the total num-ber of cocaine-exposed infants born annually to a cost estimate of more than $100 million per year for special education to address their learning and language problems. In a six-year longitudinal study of 425 inner-city children beginning at birth, Linda Mayes, a Yale psychiatrist, reports that at age four and a half the cocaine-exposed children had more trouble fo-cusing and blocking out distractions and were more impulsive than peers with otherwise similar backgrounds.[25]

Crack cocaine carries especially pernicious obstetrical risks. Unlike alcohol and other substances, legal and illegal, which can produce birth defects by derailing fetal development during the first three months, co-caine exerts much of its most devastating damage in the third trimester. A stimulant, cocaine can cause premature labor by precipitating uterine contractions—indeed, it is common street wisdom that cocaine can help a woman induce abortion. Cocaine is absorbed into the fetus's circulatory system and constricts blood vessels, which can lead to stroke in the fetus. Through surges in blood pressure, cocaine can cause the placenta to detach from the wall of the uterus, resulting in life-threatening hemorrhage to both the baby and the mother. This complication, called placental abruption, occurs in about 1 percent of the general obstetrical population but may reach 15 percent in cocaine abusers.[26]

How many women and babies are at risk for these problems? Estimates range widely from a low of 45,000 per year to 375,000. The lower number, derived from the federal National Pregnancy Health Study, is based on self-reporting and thus is probably an underestimation. The higher number is from hospital medical records of babies born with cocaine in their systems, but these hospitals were in areas of heavy drug use. An accurate number is somewhere in between.

It is true that most babies of cocaine-using mothers are born normal, but the real problem is that their odds of staying healthy, physically and psychologically, diminish precipitously after birth. "The crack baby problem is basically a pediatric one," explains Harold Pollack of the University of Michigan School of Public Health. "Most pregnant women who use drugs will have basically healthy babies. The issue is that they can't take care of them when they get home. That's why pediatricians generally take a somewhat harder line on a substance abusing woman than other health care providers."[27] Indeed, pediatricians realize that the harm to which chronic cocaine-using mothers subject their children arises out of behaviors that did not begin with pregnancy and will not end with delivery. That is why all states require physicians to report suspected child abuse, some even holding them liable for failure to report or suspect the abuse.

When Drug Addicts Have Children

One shouldn't make the leap, the bioethicist Mary Faith Marshall told a reporter, that "because a woman is a substance abuser, she is, therefore, a bad mother."[28] Mother Dog, the newsletter columnist, would agree with Marshall, but ample data contradict them.

- Children whose parents abuse drugs and alcohol are over four times more likely to be neglected than children with sober parents.[29]

- Forty percent of confirmed cases of child maltreatment involve the use of alcohol or other drugs.[30]

- Children exposed prenatally to illicit drugs are two to three times as likely to be abused or neglected as those who were not.[31]

- Cases involving parental drug addiction are characterized by repeated reports from welfare agencies.[32]

Furthermore, parental neglect often leads to sexual and physical abuse by other adults such as the mother's boyfriends. Parents leave their infants and children unattended when they go out to find drugs or sequester themselves in the bathroom or in their car to get high. During those times when parents are not around to protect them, children may be molested.[33] Still, Lawrence J. Nelson, the ethicist-lawyer, insists that the child welfare system "ought not to assume that [all drug-using] mothers are unfit."[34]

Judy Howard of the UCLA School of Medicine, who ran an outpatient treatment program, found that every one of the infants whose mothers did not cease drug use during the course of a fifteen-month observation period "showed insecure attachment demonstrated by a variety of behaviors including avoidance, fear and anger toward their mothers." She adds, "Such an extraordinarily high percentage of insecure attachments has only been previously seen in abused and neglected children."[35] By comparison, a lower, albeit still discouraging, 30 percent of children of poor mothers who did not use drugs displayed weak bonding.

Even mothers who wish to protect their children are often disturbingly naive. One addict told researchers that when "she had a hit of crack, she'd just take another vitamin pill, figuring this would balance out the effect of the hit." Another told them that she would eat a lot of white bread before smoking crack. "You know, like Wonder Bread," she said. "I figured all that bread would stop up the passage through the umbilical cord so the crack wouldn't get through to the baby."[36]

Many experts urge that children be removed from the home if their parents continue to abuse drugs. "On their own, most true addicts simply cannot take adequate care of their children. Without societal intervention, their children are condemned to lives of severe deprivation and, often, violent assault," writes Douglas J. Besharov, a child welfare specialist at the American Enterprise Institute.[37] In his book *When Drug Addicts Have Children,* he compiles the views of more than two dozen researchers, clinicians, program administrators and government officials.[38] They are nearly unanimous in calling for rapid termination of parental rights if substance abuse continues.

In interviews with more than nine hundred child welfare professionals, the researchers at Columbia University found that 82 percent believe that repeated abuse should prompt termination of parental rights.[39] Given the popularity of family preservation among social service workers, this represents a profound shift in attitude. The report concludes that abused or neglected children should be removed from the home for permanent adoption if parents who mistreat them fail to engage in treatment and to stop using drugs.

Those advocates who insist that addicts are fit enough to be parents abruptly change their minds about the limits of competence when it suits their political message. Consider the decision that Barbara Harris of Stanton, California, places before them. Harris offers addicted women $200 if they will undergo sterilization (which could be a reversible tubal ligation) or $50 if they will obtain sustained-release hormonal birth control, like Depo-Provera, which lasts three months, or Norplant, which lasts five years. Her organization, CRACK (Children Requiring a Caring Kommunity), was started in 1994 and is financed by private donations.

Harris's program has been harshly criticized by the ACLU and Planned Parenthood. "The essence of this campaign is profound hatred against poor people," says Ethel Long-Scott of the Women's Economic Agenda Project.[40] CRACK's practices are unethical, Long-Scott and others contend, because the women, lured by money or addled by drugs, cannot truly give informed consent. If that were so, why is it that these critics consider the women sufficiently equipped to raise a child?

As of the summer of 1999, Harris had paid 57 women who had been pregnant a total of 423 times. "They had 161 abortions and gave birth 262 times," Harris told the *New York Times*.[41] "Forty of those babies died and 175 are in foster care." Harris, who is white, shrugs off charges that her program is racist because the billboards announcing her offer ("If you are addicted to drugs—get birth control—get $200") are located primarily in minority neighborhoods in Florida, Minnesota and Illinois. "Don't minority babies matter?" she asked me.[42]

What's more, nearly half of the women she has paid are white. Harris's own husband is black, as are the four children the couple adopted from the same crack-using woman. "Here's this irresponsible woman walking around having babies yearly . . . and she has no intention of raising them," Harris said of the mother of her adopted kids, a woman who personifies the individual CRACK wants to reach.

The Myth of the Willing Lightbulb

The doctors and nurses at the Medical University of South Carolina did not embrace the harm reduction philosophy, nor did they see value in thinking of women as victims. It was better to view them as patients who could improve with treatment even if that treatment had to be imposed on them. The idea that patients can do well with treatment even if they don't want it does not jibe with popular understanding, which is well captured by the familiar joke: How many psychiatrists does it take to change a lightbulb? Answer: Only one, but the bulb has to want to change.

Many clinicians believe, mistakenly, that a patient must desire drug treatment in order to benefit from it, that she must first "hit bottom" and that she must want to undertake treatment for herself and not because of any outside pressure.

But addicts are notoriously poor self-disciplinarians. Most are extremely ambivalent about giving up drugs, in spite of all the damage that drugs have caused them. Addicts' problems of self-governance demand that a rehabilitative regime include limit-setting, consistency and sometimes physical containment. Paula Keller's experience captures this well.

"When I ran an outpatient program," she tells me, "only two women in four years showed up voluntarily. One of them dropped out after one week and the other lasted three weeks."

Most addicts admit that they were pressured into treatment by external forces such as employment demands, social relationships or financial conflicts. Only a small minority of addicts in treatment enrolled solely on their own personal initiative, unpressured by others.[43] Women in a focus group sponsored by the General Accounting Office noted that, "although they were forced into treatment by the state, once in treatment they gradually grew more receptive to the messages until they finally reached the point of seeking and accepting responsibility for their recovery."[44]

Coercion helped Malissa Ann Crawley of Anderson, South Carolina. In 1991 Crawley and her newborn son, Antwon, tested positive for cocaine. She was charged with unlawful neglect three weeks later, pleaded guilty and was given a five-year suspended sentence. Crawley was placed on probation, a condition of which was participation in drug treatment. During Crawley's probation her counselor reported that she had frequent positive urines. The next year Crawley gave birth to a girl. Mother and daughter tested positive for cocaine, and Crawley was again indicted on a charge of unlawful neglect.

A judge dismissed the charge, but Crawley was soon in trouble again for attacking her drug-dealer boyfriend with a knife, a violation of probation. It was only after her probation was revoked because of the knife-wielding incident and she faced jail time that Crawley stopped using drugs. She finally landed in jail in 1998 for the violation and served several months. But once released, she reentered the community drug-free and employed.

Both her ACLU lawyer and Bob Herbert, the *New York Times* columnist, condemned the "crack mom" policy, as it has been called, for taking Crawley—whose parenting skills they praised—away from her children.[45] But the South Carolina prosecutor Catherine Christophillis has a different appraisal. "After giving birth to two cocaine babies, testing positive on virtually every drug test subsequent to her initial arrest, and breaking probation by knifing a known drug dealer, she successfully kicked the habit only when told that she faced a jail sentence because of her repeated offenses," Christophillis says. "It is ironic that Malissa Crawley, whose case has been cited as an example of the program's inhumanity, is the best example I know of its success."[46]

From my own experience treating drug addicts, I know how helpful outside coercion can be in making treatment work. The patient and I do not have to waste time bargaining over how many drug tests she can fail before she pays the consequences. I do not have to risk straining the treatment relationship, since I'm not the one who makes up and enforces the rules. Instead, with externally imposed limits and expectations, I am the patient's ally. We work together to develop strategies to resist temptation because we both know there are consequences for failing, but the ultimate goal is to discover larger reasons to stay clean. What are some of these larger reasons? Family, work, respect, autonomy. Here is what my patients tell me.

> ANGELA R.: I want to have my children respect me again. They know that when I said, "Mommy has to go to the store," or, "Mommy will be in the bathroom for a while," that I was getting high. I was fooling myself to think they didn't know. And now my own authority with them is shot. How can I expect them to be honest with me and get them to listen when I tell them not to be running the streets?

> JOSEPH S.: I want my own place, my own things. Some privacy. It's been two years in and out of shelters or sleeping on friends' couches or floors. I'm sick of that. I want to have a place where my daughter can come and visit me and it's not humiliating for both of us that her father has nothing to show for himself.

> YVONNE F.: I want to go to art school. And in my spare time I want to keep working on the tattoo designs I've made. For a while I was becoming a really popular skin artist in New Orleans, but then I had to sell my equipment when I started using heroin again. I want to make enough money to buy the equipment again. I'd love to get a degree in fine arts. Painting is my passion. I can bring you some photos next week if you want to see pictures of my work.

No matter how much treatment we provide, some addicts simply will not take advantage of it. The good news is that data consistently show that treatment, *when completed,* is quite effective in achieving abstinence. Those who do enter a program voluntarily rarely complete it; about half drop out in the first three months, and 80 to 90 percent have left by the end of the first year. Among such dropouts, relapse within a year is the rule.[47]

Numerous studies demonstrate that addicts who get treatment through court order or employer mandates benefit as much as, and sometimes more than, their counterparts who enter treatment voluntarily. This is because they are less likely to drop out of treatment, according to a report from the National Institute on Drug Addiction titled "Treatment for Drug-Exposed Women and Their Children."[48] In one large-sample study, Barbara Lex at McLean Hospital in Boston examined data for five hundred women mandated to treatment by a civil judge of Massachusetts in 1995. The committed group stayed in treatment an average of four times longer than a demographically similar group of women who were voluntarily admitted.[49]

The reason sanctions and incentives can work is that the compulsion to take drugs does not necessarily dominate an addict's minute-to-minute or even day-to-day existence. Almost all addicts are capable of reflection and purposeful behavior for some, perhaps a good deal, of the time. During the course of a heroin addict's day, she may feel calm and her thoughts may be lucid so long as she is confident of access to drugs and she is using them in doses adequate to prevent withdrawal but not large enough to be sedating. Likewise, there are periods in a cocaine addict's week when she is neither engaged in a binge nor racked with intense craving for the drug. At these moments she is not controlled by a "chronic and relapsing brain disease"—the medical mantra introduced in the mid-1990s by the federal National Institute on Drug Abuse—and she might even choose to change her behavior, depending on what is at stake.

This potential for self-control permits society to entertain and enforce expectations of addicts that would never be possible for someone who had a *real* chronic and relapsing brain disease—for example, multiple sclerosis, epilepsy or schizophrenia. Making such demands is, of course, no guarantee that they will be met. But the legitimacy of such demands would encourage a range of policy and therapeutic options, using consequences and coercion, that are incompatible with the idea of a no-fault brain disease.

A major problem with coercive policies is a shortage of treatment programs in which to place addicts. For liability reasons, some programs will not accept pregnant women. Once the child is born, many residential programs will not allow the child to stay with the mother. The policy of some programs to allow only one child is better, of course, but still poses an obstacle for women who do not have reliable relatives with whom to leave their older children. Months in a residential program away from all or some of their children can be so distracting to some women as to jeopardize their treatment. Moreover, it is best to have the children present so that the mother can strengthen family bonds. Thus, adequate treatment capacity is a very important matter, but the claim by women's advocates that the only "true crisis" of the crack-mother-and-baby saga is a lack of treatment is a dangerous half-truth.

The Deterrence Debate

Once someone who abuses drugs is under the surveillance of the social service or criminal justice agencies, it becomes easier to apply leverage. Sanctions and incentives can be defined, and compliance with treatment can be overseen. Ideally, of course, a woman decides that she wants treatment and participates voluntarily. But what about the pregnant woman who is too afraid to seek help because she fears that simply showing up at a clinic will get her reported to authorities?

The risk that pregnant women may be deterred from seeking prenatal care or substance abuse treatment if they fear being arrested or losing custody of their children is a logical concern of policy proponents and critics alike.[50] The Center for Reproductive Law and Policy cites surveys of women who said that fear of being arrested or losing their children, and even a reluctance to be scolded by doctors and nurses, were barriers to seeking treatment. These claims, however, must be taken with a grain of salt. Any recovered addict will tell you that his ambivalence about giving up drugs or alcohol was once so great that virtually any excuse to forgo drug treatment—from bad weather to a headache—would have been sufficient "reason" not to get help that day.

The only evidence of avoidance that I could locate was a 1990 report from the General Accounting Office stating that "hospital officials told us that some women are now delivering their infants at home in order to prevent the state from discovering their drug use." The GAO report, while anecdotal, is a matter of concern. Fortunately, hard data from the South Carolina Department of Health and Environmental Control (DHEC) reveal a more sanguine picture.[51] In Charleston and Greenville the fraction of live births occurring outside the hospital among all minority women actually diminished somewhat from 1989 to 1994 (the years when the Medical University of South Carolina policy was in place). In Charleston out-of-hospital births totaled 1.4 percent in 1989, 2 percent in 1990, and less than 1 percent in the remaining years. Greenville had 1.3 percent out-of-hospital births in 1989, and less than 1 percent thereafter.

Thus, women were not having their babies in the streets, as had been feared. Nor did they stay away from prenatal care. In fact, most of the 119 women seen in the emergency room were not deterred from obtaining prenatal care; they never sought it in the first place.[52] In 1989 roughly 5 percent of all minority women in Charleston failed to get prenatal care. The next year the percentage was 5.5, and thereafter it hovered around 3. In Greenville as well, about 4 percent of minority women had no prenatal care in 1989; subsequently it was about 3 percent (DHEC data).

The Charleston experience is reminiscent of the example of mandatory HIV reporting. As of November 1, 1999, thirty-four states had implemented a system of name-based reporting of HIV infection. Rightly, the question of whether this practice affected individuals' willingness to seek testing and care was examined by the Centers for Disease Control. After looking at whether HIV testing patterns changed after reporting policies went into effect, the agency concluded that it has no such effect.[53] In one nine-state survey the CDC interviewed roughly twenty-three hundred untested but at-risk individuals and asked why they had not yet been tested for HIV. The most common reply—given by 25 percent of the sample—was fear of learning they were positive. By contrast, only 2 percent said that having their name reported was the primary reason for avoiding the test.[54]

This does not prove, of course, that in South Carolina some women did not stay away from a prenatal clinic because of the risk of being reported. Similarly, there may be mothers who don't bring their abused children to the pediatrician for fear of being reported. But to my knowledge, there is little published information on whether or not fewer pregnant women actually sought care in the wake of more restrictive policies. One survey of ten hospitals across the country found that 29 to 70 percent of women using drugs did not get adequate prenatal care, depending on the hospital, compared with 8 to 35 percent who did not use drugs: it is simply not a priority for most women who are heavy drug users.[55] Asking women, as surveys do, whether, in principle, they would stay away from treatment if they could be prosecuted and jailed for using drugs is irrelevant to current practice. South Carolina and other states impose only compulsory treatment, not criminal penalties and incarceration, and do so only after several attempts to become drug-free have failed. Not surprisingly, officials like William J. Domina of the district attorney's office in Waukesha County, Wisconsin, are frustrated with the advocates. "By continually mischaracterizing the Wisconsin law [for compulsory treatment] the extremists spread the fear they criticize the law for generating," Mr. Domina says.[56]

At Leigh Beasley's clinic in Pickens County, in a hardscrabble part of northwestern South Carolina, there seems to be little problem with deterrence. The data even suggest that being held responsible may encourage women to get treatment. Of all women who delivered live babies in 1989 (the year testing began), 65 to 70 percent entered care during the first trimester. That proportion steadily rose, to 73 percent in 1991, 80 percent in 1994 and almost 84 percent in 1997. Over the same period the portion of women whose prenatal care was inadequate, as defined by widely accepted standards, fell 21 percent. "Our testing certainly did not have a negative effect on coming in for prenatal care," says clinic charge nurse Trish Locklair. According to her log on "late entries"—women who do not start coming in for care until the second or third trimester—even those who used drugs denied that they put off care because of a fear of being reported.[57]

Safe Havens

Beasley's Pickens County clinic is one place that's getting it right. Her brightly lit clinic, which I visited in 1998, serves primarily poor white families. Pregnant women in Pickens County who use drugs are more likely to use marijuana than cocaine. In Greenville, about forty miles away, the poor population is predominantly black and pregnant women are more likely to use crack.

All pregnant women are asked to give a voluntary urine sample for drug testing when they begin prenatal visits at the Pickens County clinic. Reporting a positive test or reporting a woman's refusal to take a test to child protective services is not mandatory until after the twenty-third week of pregnancy. The clinic has an excellent record of cooperation. In the first ten years of testing, which was initiated in 1989, only one woman refused. Urine testing is critical because a substantial minority of drug-using women deny doing drugs. In one study, 24 percent of women who used cocaine would have been missed if the clinic had relied solely on self-report.[58] Rather, Beasley's patients are willing to disclose use, but, the doctor confirmed, "we would have missed nineteen women in 1998 if we did not do testing."[59]

If a woman tests positive in the first twenty-three weeks, she is referred to substance abuse counseling with Jo Ann Musto Brink, who says that her goal is to "help the women get drug-free before giving birth."[60] She usually succeeds. "The women all talk to each other, and they know that our goal is to help them, not to get them in trouble with the law," Brink says. Of the seventy-four women who tested positive in 1998 for marijuana, cocaine or heroin, only two went on to have babies who tested positive; one of those babies was placed in protection agency custody.

Brenda Cummings, one of Brink's patients, got married for the first time at age fourteen and had her first child at fifteen. She used alcohol and marijuana for the next decade and a half. At age thirty she came to the clinic twelve weeks pregnant. She was smoking marijuana regularly, and despite the urging of clinic staff, she didn't stop. Finally Brink made it clear to Cummings that if she didn't quit by her sixth month, there would be serious consequences. The child protection agency "got me scared," Cummings tells me. "I didn't have a choice but to quit. I couldn't lose my kids. Did it seem like punishment? Yes, but the Lord gave us children, and we're the ones who have to take care of them. I was forced to use my willpower. I'm not sure I would have done that without Jo Ann."[61] Cummings's daughter Margaret was born healthy and drug-free and lives with Cummings and her new husband.

Brink's patients often need more than drug treatment. Without job skills or a high school diploma, these women, even if they stay clean, will almost inevitably remain on public assistance. Paula Keller runs Serenity Place, a residential program for young mothers in Greenville. Thirty-two-year-old Kiva Greer, a resident I interviewed in 1999, had no intention of quitting drugs when she came in. "I thought I'd come in here and play around and tell them what they wanted to hear," she says.[62] For the past decade she had been in and out of drug treatment clinics for problems with marijuana and alcohol; five years before she had begun using crack. Two of her children, ages eight and twelve, live with relatives; her two- and three-year-old sons are with her at Serenity Place.

When "Noodle," her youngest son, was born, Greer was using marijuana. The hospital notified the child protective agency, and she was told that if she didn't stop she'd risk losing two of her other children and going to jail. "What choice do you really have?" she asks. "I took Serenity Place. I didn't want to give up Noodle." When did she decide to take the program seriously? "I'd never been in a residence before. It took about three weeks. I mean, you're around people all the time, you can't get away with too much. And I saw how well the other women were doing, how they were getting it together, getting jobs or going back to school. That's what I want. Maybe a career in fashion merchandising."

Often the women are so ill prepared to be mothers, Keller says, that a major focus of the program is simply helping them to develop self-discipline. Without the regimentation of the daily routine, Keller says, many of the women would "feed their kids candy for breakfast or lay in bed most of the day."[63] Teaching them how and when to discipline their children is also important, Keller explains. Three-quarters of her referrals are from prenatal clinics like Beasley's, neonatal nurseries and the County Health Department—further evidence that women are not staying away en masse from medical services. "When I first heard about the policy," Leigh Beasley tells me, "I was very uneasy. I was afraid it could scare women away. But now I'm a great supporter when I see how many women and children were helped."[64]

The Whitner Case:
Supreme Court Versus Anti-Mother

Back in Charleston, in the southern end of the state, the Medical University had suspended its drug testing policy in 1994, after the Office of Civil Rights stepped in. But in 1998 a modified drug testing policy was reinstated. The new policy involves law enforcement authorities only after a woman has refused multiple offers of help and evaded several layers of supervision from child protection authorities. Should the mother-to-be refuse to cooperate with treatment, the state child protection agency petitions family court for authority to intervene.

The intervention is often commitment to a residential treatment program. No women have gone to jail.[65] Yet the debate over the privacy rights of women who use drugs in the late stages of pregnancy remains vigorous and far more attentive to questions about whether the policy is "good for women" or "good for African Americans" than to what is best for the children or even for the addicts themselves.

The Medical University was able to enact the new guidelines because of a crucial court decision: *Whitner v. State of South Carolina*. In 1990 Cornelia Whitner, then thirty-two, lost custody of both her children after she abandoned them in the midst of a crack binge. Whitner was no paragon of motherhood. At the time she had convictions for shoplifting, petty larceny, using a false name and trespassing.

A week before Christmas 1991, Whitner, seven months pregnant with her third child, came before a Pickens County judge, Frank Eppes, and pleaded guilty to neglecting her toddler, Leroy. Eppes sentenced her to probation and ordered her to stay away from drugs and alcohol. Violating those terms, he told her, would mean ten years in prison. When her son Tevin was born about seven weeks later, he tested positive for cocaine. As promised, Eppes gave Whitner ten years.

In July 1996 the South Carolina Supreme Court decided against Whitner, whose lawyers appealed the ruling that a viable fetus has legal standing as a child. The Center for Reproductive Law and Policy appealed to the U.S. Supreme Court. Among those filing friend-of-the-court briefs against the state were the American College of Obstetricians and Gynecologists, the American Nurses Association, the American Medical Women's Association and the National Association of Alcoholism and Drug Abuse Counselors. In May 1998 the justices declined to hear the appeal.

The crucial legal question settled, South Carolina's attorney general issued a statewide protocol for managing drug- or alcohol-abusing women and their newborns in all kinds of clinical settings: private or public, inpatient or outpatient, emergency room or clinic. Many organizations helped draft the state protocol, among them the South Carolina chapter of the American College of Obstetrics and Gynecology, the South Carolina Hospital Association, the South Carolina Medical Association and the South Carolina Department of Alcohol and Other Drug Abuse Services.

Not a Dangerous Place

The original Charleston policy was unnecessarily harsh: there is no medical benefit in jailing a woman who has a drug-positive baby, yet a number did spend some time incarcerated. The subsequent developments, however, have enabled South Carolina to develop a model program for steering women into treatment and their children toward more promising futures. South Carolina's program, with its combination of carrots and sticks, embodies an important clinical reality: addicts must anticipate or experience consequences if they are to alter their behavior. It also reflects a reasonable decision to accept a trade-off: the risk of deterring some women who *might* avoid prenatal care versus intervening with women whose capacity for responsible parenthood is already clearly in doubt. After all, even after suffering obstetrical complications or delivering a drug-positive baby, these women remain at high risk of continuing to use drugs after they take the baby home from the hospital.

Clearly, authorities can act to diminish the coercive aspects of the program by mounting an educational campaign informing women that simply showing up for care, even if they use drugs, does not get them in trouble with the law. In fact, the aid of women already in the program is a big help to Paula Keller. "Their peers tell the women how important it is to come into Serenity Place and how much it helped them," she says.

This isn't "pitting" the fetus against the mother, as Lynn Paltrow worries.[66] A *Time* magazine piece proclaimed South Carolina "a dangerous place for pregnant women who abuse drugs." In truth, the state is one of the safest places for them and their children. Incarceration is now a rare outcome for women who are far more likely to enjoy the vast benefit of programs like Keller's Serenity Place. That is not punitive; it is the prescription of choice for changing the behavior of addicts who find themselves locked in a cycle of self-destruction.

6

Race and Medicine

ONE EVENING IN 1994 Dr. Pius K. Kamau was on call at his Denver hospital when a nineteen-year-old car crash victim was admitted to the intensive-care unit coughing up blood. The young man, a white supremacist skinhead sporting a swastika tattoo, was shocked to look up from his bed and see Kamau, a black man, taking care of him. The patient refused to have anything to do with his doctor. "He never talked to me directly; all of our dealings were via white nurses," Kamau writes. "They interpreted to him what I said, as if I spoke in another language. He never allowed his open eyes to rest on mine again."[1]

Despite the difficulties, Kamau did his work and the patient recovered. The doctor had fulfilled the Hippocratic ideal to which he was sworn: being an honorable agent of the patient. Judging from the searching personal essay he wrote about the experience, I think Kamau would be deeply offended at the suggestion that a physician might compromise his standard of care for patients such as this hate-filled nineteen-year-old.

According to new conventional wisdom, however, it takes far less than an insufferably bigoted patient to cause a physician to lower his standard of treatment. A mismatch in race between doctor and patient—especially when the doctor is white and the patient is not—may be enough to trigger subtle, or not so subtle, biases that result in second-rate medical treatment and poorer health. "It is increasingly evident that African-Americans and other minority patients have strong grounds for doubting both the goodwill and the color blindness of White medical practitioners," writes Kenneth DeVille of the Department of Medical Humanities at the East Carolina University School of Medicine.[2] No less authoritative a voice than the American Medical Association's official newspaper has claimed that "a growing body of research reports that racial disparities in health status can be explained, at least in part, by racism and discrimination within the health care system itself."[3] This is why, according to the Reverend Al Sharpton, health will be the "new civil rights battlefront," a prediction echoed by other black leaders, including the Reverend Jesse Jackson, NAACP chairman Julian Bond and the Congressional Black Caucus.[4]

In a 1998 radio address delivered during Black History Month, President Clinton spoke of race and health. "Nowhere are the divisions of race and ethnicity more sharply drawn than in the health of our people."[5] It is indeed true that black Americans are less healthy than whites and Asians on a number of measures, such as life expectancy, infant mortality and death from cancer. This often remains true even when insurance coverage is taken into account.[6] Beyond these facts, the president could only speculate when he said that perhaps one of the reasons for racial disparities is "discrimination in the delivery of health services."[7]

Given the history of systematic racial discrimination and segregation in the health care system, lingering bias seems, at first, plausible. Black patients were treated on separate and inferior hospital wards—a policy that persisted at many hospitals in the Deep South until the late 1960s. Once routinely barred from joining hospital staffs and medical societies, black physicians started their own institutions to treat other blacks who were denied adequate care by the white-controlled medical facilities.[8] As late as the mid-1960s several medical schools had restrictions against admitting black students.[9]

A particularly appalling episode in medical research was the Tuskegee Syphilis Study, whose purpose was to study the natural progression of the disease in black men. In the notorious "experiment," which lasted from 1932 to 1972, roughly four hundred black men in the late stages of syphilis were never told of their condition, never given any kind of treatment and never warned about transmitting it—grossly unethical practices that would never be tolerated today.

Decades later, however, accusations of medical bias still linger. According to Vanessa Northington Gamble, a physician and vice president of Community and Minority Programs at the Association of American Medical Colleges, "Tuskegee symbolizes for many African-Americans the racism that pervades American institutions, including the medical profession."[10] In the fall of 1999 the U.S. Commission on Civil Rights informed Congress and the White House that "racism continue[s] to infect" the health care system.[11] Earlier that year an official of the Association of American Medical Colleges commented on physicians' unwitting biases. "Most doctors think they are fair," he told the *Boston Globe*. "That they carry bias is very hard for them to think about."[12]

For her part, Leslie Pickering Francis, a medical ethicist at the University of Utah, prefers to believe that "racism [is] the presumptive cause of . . . health care problems minorities face" until there is evidence to the contrary.[13] This view is increasingly common—not too surprising considering the habit nowadays of presuming that discrimination inevitably lies beneath the surface of any race-related difference in social outcome. But evidence suggests that many race-related differences in health are not what they seem to observers like Professor Francis, Reverend Sharpton and the Commission on Civil Rights.

The charge of physician bias against minority patients is often made reflexively, overlooking the myriad complicated reasons for differences in care. In this chapter I present evidence that supports other interpretations of "health disparities," as they are often called.[14] As we will see, the race-related differences that do exist in both access to health care and in health status are better understood—and remedied—from the vantage points of clinical need and health care financing—not race politics.

Do Physicians Treat Minority Patients Differently?

A study in the *New England Journal of Medicine* in 1999 described differences in the treatment of lung cancer between black and white patients who were beneficiaries of Medicare insurance.[15] In a careful analysis, Peter B. Bach and his colleagues at Memorial Sloan-Kettering Cancer Center in New York City looked at the records of more than ten thousand patients who received diagnoses of operable lung cancer. Seventy-seven percent of the white patients underwent surgery compared with 64 percent of the black patients. Five years after diagnosis, only one-quarter of black patients were still alive compared to one-third of whites.

What accounts for the different rates of surgery? Did doctors not suggest the treatment as often to their black patients, or did these patients more often refuse the recommendation for surgery? Were the black patients more likely to have poor lung function, such as more carbon dioxide buildup, or other problems that would have prohibited surgery or contributed to earlier demise? Details like these are crucial in explaining why surgery was used less for black patients and why death rates differed, but those were not the questions that Bach and his colleagues set out to answer.[16] Indeed, the authors themselves said they could not offer an explanation for different rates of surgery based on the kinds of data they collected.

Other physicians, however, were ready with hypotheses. "Possibly, physicians are treating cancer patients not just based upon their illness and recommended treatment, but on the basis of their race," suggested Dr. Hugh Stallworth of the American Cancer Society.[17] A more emphatic reaction greeted a report in the *Annals of Emergency Medicine* that 74 percent of white patients with fractures of the extremities received pain medication in the emergency room compared with 57 percent of black patients.[18] "I think it's racism, flat out," said Dr. Lewis Goldfrank, director of emergency services at Bellevue Hospital in New York City.[19]

Responses like these would probably not surprise John Landsverk of Children's Hospital in San Diego. As he observes: "The usual implication of such disparities [in treatment rates] is that the health care system is biased against persons of the ethnic minority group and that the bias is likely to be found even in professional clinicians' perceptions of clinical problems and [referrals for] clinical procedures."[20]

In light of this, Landsverk is especially enthusiastic about one study led by a group of doctors from the University of Pittsburgh that found no race-related differences in the treatment of children with behavioral problems.[21] Their report appeared in the journal *Medical Care* one month after

Bach's study, but it attracted little public attention. It should have: it was "an important nonfinding," as Landsverk notes in an accompanying editorial in the same journal. Not only did the Pittsburgh study include a very large sample—almost fifteen thousand children treated in clinics across the country and Canada—but most important, the researchers interviewed the parent and doctor of *every* patient. The results: the race and ethnicity of the child had no relationship to clinician patterns of drug prescribing, referral or diagnosis of behavioral problems. The clinicians also reported spending slightly *more* time with minority children than with their white counterparts.

The handful of studies just discussed gives a taste of the challenges inherent in interpreting health disparities data. First, the vast majority of treatment disparity studies are what scientists call "retrospective." That is, the raw data already exist in hospital records, and researchers use them (in retrospect) to explore a specific question. (For example, are there more visits to emergency rooms on nights with a full moon?) The disadvantage of this approach is that key questions cannot be asked directly of the very people being studied: for example, in the case of the lung cancer study, did subjects want or refuse a specific treatment? Did their physicians offer it, and if not, why? Second, as Landsverk's reaction to the University of Pittsburgh study suggests, the *absence* of alleged racial bias does not make news. Consider the following example of a study that made a media splash the first time around.

A Misdiagnosed Case of Physician Bias

Cardiac catheterization is a procedure used to discern whether there is blockage in the coronary arteries—the vessels that feed blood to the heart itself—and thus whether the patient is at risk for a heart attack. The delicate process involves introducing a catheter into an artery in the leg and threading it upward toward the heart. When it reaches the point near the apex of the heart where the coronary arteries branch off, dye is squirted in, and the arterial patterns show up on a real-time X-ray. This is generally the first step in determining whether the vessels can be opened wider using a tiny balloon (balloon angioplasty) or whether some or all of the vessels must be replaced in a bypass operation.

Struck by the observation that black patients undergo catheterization less often than whites, Dr. Kevin A. Schulman and others at Georgetown University Medical Center wanted to examine how doctors make their decisions to refer patients for the procedure.[22] The researchers recruited 720 general internists at medical conventions and asked them to participate in a study of clinical decisionmaking. The internists were not told that a primary purpose of the study was to explore how the race and sex of the patient might affect those decisions, nor that the researchers expected to find that African Americans (and women) would be referred for cardiac catheterization less frequently than white men.

The doctors watched a video of actors wearing hospital gowns and answering questions posed to them by an interviewer who elicited their complaints about chest pain and other relevant medical and personal history. The viewing doctors were informed of the actor-patients' insurance types and their occupations. All the questions asked of the actors and their responses, down to the gestures they used in describing their symptoms, were scripted to minimize inconsistencies. As a group, the doctors, most of whom were white, viewed 144 different videotapes, one for every possible combination of race (black or white), sex (male or female) and age (fifty-five and seventy years old), and including differing clinical variables, like the nature of the chest pain and EKG and stress test results. Individual doctors were shown one randomly selected video.

Next, the physicians were asked whether the patients' complaints appeared to reflect heart disease or another kind of distress, such as indigestion, and to rate the likelihood that the pain was indeed heart-related. As it turned out, all eight actor-patients received similar ratings from the doctors, leading the authors to assume the doctors would refer for catheterization at similar rates as well. Yet this did not happen; according to Schulman, "women and blacks [in the study] were less likely to be referred for cardiac catheterization than men and whites." Doctors did not refer white men about 9 percent of the time, while the black actor-patients and women of both races did not get referred 15 percent of the time. If representative of actual clinical outcomes, Schulman told the media, this would mean that blacks are "40 percent less likely to be referred for cardiac catheterization compared to whites."[23] He misspoke, however: what it really would mean is that white patients have a 40 percent lower chance of *not* being referred. Quite a difference, as we will see.

These findings were presented in an article titled "The Effect of Race and Sex on Physicians' Recommendations for Cardiac Catheterization," published in the *New England Journal of Medicine* in February 1999. Schulman and his associates speculate:

> Our finding that the race and sex of the patient influence the recommendations of physicians independently of other factors may suggest bias on the part of the physicians. However, our study could not assess the form of bias. Bias may represent overt prejudice on the part of physicians or, more likely, could be the result of subconscious perceptions rather than deliberate actions or thoughts. Subconscious bias occurs when a patient's membership in a target group automatically activates a cultural stereotype in the physician's memory regardless of the level of prejudice the physician has.[24]

The study was a media sensation. On ABC's *World News This Morning,* Juju Chang told viewers: "How your doctor treats your heart may depend on the color of your skin. . . . The bias shows up in the diagnosis, and doctors don't even realize it."[25] Peter Jennings predicted that the study would make "political waves" because it showed that "prejudice among doctors causes a gap in the quality of health care between blacks and whites."[26]

On *Nightline,* Ted Koppel set up the story like this: "Last night we told you how the town of Jasper, Texas, is coming to terms with being the place where a black man was dragged to his death behind a truck by an avowed racist. Tonight we're going to focus on [doctors] . . . who would be shocked to learn that what they do routinely fits quite easily into the category of racist behavior."[27] Newspaper headlines echoed the theme:

"Cardiac Testing: Study Finds Women, Blacks Are Being Shortchanged," the *Chicago Tribune* said.[28] "Health Care: It's Better If You're White," announced *The Economist*.[29] And all the articles repeated Schulman's claim that blacks were 40 percent less likely to be referred.

Some of the most intense—indeed, self-flagellating—reactions came from the medical profession itself. An editorial in the *Lancet*, Britain's foremost medical journal, saw the findings as being "as close to a definition of institutionalised racism as doctors and health-care providers may dare to get."[30] Aubrey Lewis, a Long Island cardiologist, warned on *Nightline* that "if this [physician bias] continues on, you're looking at literally a decimation of the African American population."

No one seemed to notice another article, published earlier that same February in the *Annals of Internal Medicine* by the Harvard researcher Lucian L. Leape and his colleagues. In their evaluation of thirteen New York City hospitals, Leape's group found that African American patients are as likely to undergo cardiac bypass or balloon angioplasty as whites and Hispanics, and in some hospitals *more* likely to receive a recommendation for these procedures.[31]

A Second, Sober Look at Schulman's Study

A careful look at the work of Schulman and his colleagues reveals a number of intriguing things. One is the doctors' impressions of the subjects: one might be surprised to learn that they found the *white* actor-patients to be the least agreeable. When asked, for example, to rate their impressions of the subjects' personal characteristics, the doctors rated the white men as more "hostile" and gave them the lowest ratings on scales that ranged from "ignorant" (lowest score) to "knowledgeable" (highest score) and from "poor communicator" to "good communicator." Similarly, doctors judged white men to be more "dependent" than their black counterparts, more "sad," more "negative" in disposition, more "worried" and more "likely to over-report symptoms."

Finally, the white males were judged "most likely to sue." With such a litigious profile, one might have expected white men to be *over-referred* by physicians in order to avoid malpractice lawsuits.

The second revelation came six months after the Schulman study appeared, when the *New England Journal of Medicine* itself published a powerful rebuttal. Lisa M. Schwartz, Steven Woloshin and H. Gilbert Welch, all physicians at the White River Junction Veterans Administration Hospital in Vermont, reanalyzed Schulman's data and showed that the actual average referral rates for three of the four groups were in fact the same.[32] White men, white women and black men were all referred by nine in ten doctors. Only black women, for reasons that remain unclear, had a lower referral rate: about eight in ten. Put another way, the black women were 88 percent as likely as the white women and men of both races to be referred for catheterization in the actor-patient study.

The doctors from White River Junction also expressed dismay at what might be called the statistical sleight-of-hand that Schulman and his colleagues used to support their hypothesis of physician referral bias in favor of white men. It was only because Schulman and colleagues combined the referral rates for black men (91 percent) and black women (79 percent) to yield an 85 percent black referral rate that they could conclude that the racial differences were so marked.[33] This maneuver led to the "mistaken impression that blacks had a 40 percent lower probability of referral than whites, whereas, in fact, the probability of referral for blacks was 7 percent lower," wrote the White River Junction doctors. "These exaggerations serve only to fuel anger and undermine the trust between physicians and their patients."[34] Schwartz and her colleagues were not alone in expressing concern; the *NEJM* editors published a note in the same issue regretting that they had not required the authors to use more straightforward statistical measures. "We take responsibility for the media's overinterpretation of [this] article. . . . The evidence of racism and sexism in [the Schulman] study was overstated," the editors wrote.[35]

Nevertheless, even after seeing how his findings had been interpreted by the press and used to goad racial resentments, Schulman wouldn't budge. "Our study will . . . encourage the medical profession to seek ways to eliminate unconscious bias that may influence physicians' clinical decisions," he maintained.[36] Schulman also met with the Congressional Black Caucus at its invitation and briefed the members on bias in the health care system.[37] Also sticking with Schulman's interpretation was Paul Douglass, a cardiologist at Morehouse School of Medicine. "You can argue with statistics all day," he told *USA Today*. "We have to face the reality of our situation: there is a gender and racial bias."[38] Compared with the tidal wave of coverage triggered by the Schulman study, the article by Schwartz and her colleagues generated a mere trickle of media interest, as noted by the columnist John Leo and the media magazine *Brill's Content*.[39]

Alternative Explanations for Differences in Treatment

Less eye-catching than accusations of bias are the everyday aspects of clinical care that account for many of the recorded disparities. For example, one reason procedure rates differ is that medical problems do not necessarily occur with the same frequency across races. As a 1999 report from the Henry J. Kaiser Family Foundation points out, "It should be noted that every differential in care is not necessarily a problem and the level of care obtained by whites may not be the appropriate standard for comparison."[40] Consider these facts: uterine fibroid tumors, and thus hysterectomies, are more common in black women than in whites, while osteoporosis-related fractures, and thus hip replacements, are rarer. Limb amputation is more common among black patients, typically because thicker atherosclerosis of the blood vessels in the leg makes it harder to perform limb-saving surgery.[41]

African Americans suffer stroke at many times the rate of whites yet undergo a procedure to unclog arteries in the neck (endarterectomy) only one-fourth as often. Racism? Unlikely. Some studies have documented a greater aversion to surgery and other invasive procedures among African American patients, but the more substantial reason, in the case of endarterectomy, is clinical.[42] It turns out that whites tend to have their obstructions in the large, superficial carotid arteries of the neck region, which are readily accessible to surgery. Blacks, by comparison, tend to have their blockages in the branches of the carotids. These smaller vessels run deeper and further up into the head where the surgeon cannot reach them.[43]

Thus, even without financial obstacles, an African American patient at high risk for stroke is far less likely than a white counterpart to undergo endarterectomy. Yet indoctrinologists like David R. Williams, a sociologist at the University of Michigan's Institute for Social Research, are quick to turn this disparity into evidence of bias. After all, they argue, if money is not an issue, then the difference in treatment *must* represent bias on the part of the doctors. *American Medical News*, the newspaper of the American Medical Association, gives voice to this view: "National studies, such as one that examined care at Dept. of Veterans Affairs medical facilities—where all of the patients have comparable insurance coverage—suggest 'racial disparities in the quality of medical care do not merely reflect the behavior of a few bad apples,' Dr. Williams said. 'The evidence is too overwhelming and the pattern is too pervasive.'"[44]

Williams seems not to consider a different interpretation: the patients' clinical needs rather than the doctors' personal biases are dictating the care. Think about it: If not for concern about the patient (many of whom are treated in private hospitals and have health insurance), why wouldn't physicians perform a reimbursable procedure?

Another consideration in performing procedures is the clinical condition of the patient. Does he have other medical problems that alter the risk-to-benefit ratio of a procedure and make the outcome less favorable? The treatment of heart disease, for example, often needs to be modified in the presence of uncontrolled high blood pressure and diabetes—conditions more typical of black patients with heart disease than of their white counterparts.[45]

Then there is the site of care itself. Some hospitals simply do not offer certain cardiac procedures, such as bypass grafts or balloon angioplasty. Examining a sample taken from New York City hospitals, Dr. Lucian L. Leape of the Harvard School of Public Health and his colleagues found that about one-fifth of all patients needing these procedures do not get them, largely because those hospitals do not offer them. Leape found that failure to recommend these procedures—and hence to transfer a patient to a hospital where it could be performed—is equal across all groups of black, white and Hispanic patients.[46] Conversely, when medical care is readily available for special patient populations (for example, the veterans' affairs medical centers or the military services), racial differences in treatment and outcome can melt away. For example, veterans with colorectal and prostate cancer show no race-related differences in treatment availability, treatment methods or survival rates.[47]

Fairness and Kidney Transplantation

Patients' attitudes toward illness and care also play a role in determining the treatment they receive. The nature of their belief in their personal susceptibility to disease, the seriousness with which they perceive disease, their confidence that the treatment will work—and even that the medical system is benign—are all relevant.[48] Differences in health beliefs account for some of the reluctance in the African American community to donate (and sometimes receive) kidneys, according to Dr. Clive O. Callender, head of transplant surgery at Howard University Medical Center in Washington, DC.

Callender tells me that, compared to whites, African American patients are less trustful that they will be well cared for, whether as a living relative undergoing surgery to donate a kidney or as a patient undergoing transplantation surgery to receive one. Some fear that signing a donor card will lead to premature declaration of death.[49] Others express concern that a deceased donor will either be disfigured or unable to get into heaven without all his body parts. A potential recipient may also object on religious grounds to having the tissue of a dead person in his body. Moreover, blacks are not as likely as whites to believe that people who get transplants gain additional healthy years of life.[50]

To enhance recruitment of African American donors and dispel the myths surrounding donation, Clive Callender directs the national Minority Organ Tissue Transplantation and Education Program (MOTTEP), which operates in over a dozen cities. Understanding patients' objections to donation and demystifying the process is critical because severe (or "end-stage") renal disease is about four times more common in blacks than in whites and, as we will see, there are considerable benefits to receiving a kidney from a living donor of the same race.

To create incentives for organ donation and expand the black organ donor pool, Wayne B. Arnason, a minister writing in the *Hastings Center Report*, has proposed an experimental protocol that would try to pair a black donor kidney with a black recipient.[51] Some African Americans have expressed a desire that their organs be earmarked for black recipients.[52] Arnason's proposal addresses the fears of some black patients that they are being discriminated against in the kidney transplantation process, fears stoked by observers like David Barton Smith, a sociologist at the University of Michigan, who asserts in his 1999 book *Health Care Divided: Race and Healing a Nation:* "The assumptions that served as justification for the Tuskegee Study remain in evidence among those providing health services to [the black] population. . . . Blacks have lower rates of kidney transplants . . . even where no differences in insurance or ability to pay exist."[53]

This matter has attracted the attention of a wide spectrum of advocates, from the Reverend Louis Farrakhan (who has said that whites condone black-on-black killing as a source of transplantable organs) to law professors who propose suing the federal government for violating civil rights laws in the allocation of organs.[54] The U.S. Commission on Civil Rights has also weighed in: "Black patients remain less likely than other minorities and whites to receive a kidney transplant," it reported in 1999, calling this "an aspect of health care inequality that thus far seems to have eluded the [HHS's] Office of Civil Rights."[55]

To assess the fairness of the charges levied by the Commission on Civil Rights and others we must first walk through the steps involved in donating and receiving a kidney. The road starts at renal dialysis. Every two or three days patients with end-stage kidney disease undergo a process called renal dialysis while they wait for a kidney to become available. During the three-to-four-hour dialysis process, patients are hooked up to a machine that acts as an external kidney, removing the fluid and metabolic by-products that are normally cleared by the kidney and excreted as urine. For unclear reasons, black patients, on average, tolerate dialysis better than white patients—who are more likely than black patients to die while on the waiting list—and blacks can be maintained longer in a healthy state before transplantation.[56] Just the opposite is true, however, once the operation has taken place: black patients, on average, do not tolerate the transplanted organ as well as whites, and they must return to dialysis support sooner and more frequently.[57]

Since patients of any race remain at greater risk of new complications or even death the longer they are on dialysis, the definitive treatment is typically transplantation. Thus, it is crucial that patients be put on the waiting list as soon as possible. Yet black patients are about half as likely to be put on the list at any point in time; once listed, they remain there about twice as long as white patients until a suitable organ becomes available.[58] Thus, in 1998 the average white candidate was twice as likely to receive a kidney as his African American counterpart.[59] These differences need to be investigated and explained.

Much of the demographic and clinical data on organ transplantation come from the private nonprofit organization UNOS (United Network for Organ Sharing), which serves as part of the organ allocation system for the federal government. It coordinates the waiting list, distributes kidneys and devises complex formulas for organ allocation that take into account a patient's medical condition and other biological factors. The UNOS system also collects data on the characteristics of transplant candidates and recipients so that researchers have access to large and representative databases. What do these and other data tell us about the dynamics of kidney allocation?

They indicate that the earliest step in the long process leading to kidney transplantation—being put on the waiting list—depends on the patient having access to good health care in general. If a patient does not have a regular doctor who will refer him to a transplant center, the entire process of obtaining an organ is slowed. The center registers patients for the waiting list, determines medical suitability and conducts the pretransplant workup. Ability to pay does not seem to pose a barrier to kidney transplantation, since any patient with end-stage renal disease is eligible for public insurance that covers dialysis, medication, doctors' services and transplant surgery.[60]

Another key aspect of the transplantation process is the patient's interest in receiving a kidney. UNOS data suggest that African American patients decline the procedure more often than do whites.[61] Reports have documented that black transplant candidates were more often undecided, more apt to decline the transplant operation at the last minute, more often unavailable owing to illness and more likely to be unlocatable when a kidney became available.[62] A 1999 study by John Z. Ayanian and his colleagues at the Harvard Medical School discovered yet another pattern. In interviews with about fourteen hundred patients on dialysis, the researchers found that although black patients were somewhat less likely to express a desire for a kidney, their markedly lower rates of referral to the waiting list (a little over 50 percent for black patients versus over 70 percent for whites) could not be explained solely by this difference or by other clinical factors.[63] The Ayanian study was especially noteworthy because it was prospective: the researchers interviewed patients directly, in real time, about their preferences. The drawback to the study, however, was that the researchers did not question the doctors about their decisions to refer their patients to the waiting list. A more detailed look at the non-racial characteristics of patients who were placed on the waiting list reveals some factors that might have influenced the doctors: whether the patient was "very certain" about wanting a kidney (about seventy out of one hundred white patients were "very certain," compared to sixty out of one hundred black patients), younger age, whether the patient expected to live longer with a transplant and whether the patient reported greater agreement with the doctor's medical decisions.

Ayanian and his colleagues also found that black patients were less likely to report that a physician had discussed with them the possibility of receiving a living kidney from a family member. Similarly, Edward Guadagnoli and his colleagues, also at the Harvard Medical School, found that hospital staff at 112 hospitals approached white families of the recently deceased to request the body's organs up to twice as often as they approached black families. Apart from the obvious reason for not approaching the family—that the recently deceased was not a suitable medical candidate for donation—the authors speculate that sometimes medical personnel *presume* that black families will decline since their rates of refusal, when asked, are known to be higher.[64] It is also possible that differences in manifestations of grief influence the decision to approach a family. Personnel, for example, are more reluctant to approach families who seem extremely traumatized by their loved one's death because it might seem cruel to compound their distress.[65]

Thus, the remedy for recruiting more organ donors is better education of both medical personnel and the public. Medical personnel, research indicates, have better success at requesting donation when they are more skilled at meeting families' informational and emotional needs.[66] A number of variables have been shown to influence willingness to donate a loved one's organs, among them the belief that the loved one received the best possible care. In addition, families are more likely to donate when they understand the concept of brain death (and have discussed it *before* the request for an organ is made), if they are given enough time to make an informed decision, if procedures are described in understandable language and if the discussion takes place in a quiet and private place.[67]

Combining these principles with better education for the public through a program like Clive Callender's MOTTEP seems most promising. Simply getting more people to have a family discussion about donation is important because families are more likely to agree to the donation process if they know the deceased had previously expressed a desire to give his organs. The MOTTEP program also involves explaining the biology of matching and the nature of the surgical procedure, and working with churches to dispel religion-based myths. Callender's results are encouraging: by the late 1990s, 45 percent of kidneys transplanted at Howard University (a predominantly African American institution) were from black donors; a decade earlier the figure had been under 20 percent.

Fairness Continued

Now let us turn to the clinical aspects of transplantation. A crucial dimension is tissue compatibility. Without a good "match," the donor kidney will provoke the recipient's immune system to attack or "reject" it. The better the match on biological variables, the better the outcome. According to a report issued by the UNOS Histocompatibility Committee, black patients in need of a transplant wait longer owing to factors such as blood type, sensitization and some antigens.[68] Similarly, Rand researchers found that "once a patient is on the waiting list, biological factors may predominate" in explaining his lower chances of receiving a kidney.[69]

A technique called antigen matching is used to test for different combinations of six major antigens, or proteins, found on the surface of tissues. A perfect six-out-of-six match is the ideal condition for compatibility between donor and recipient. A complete match is far less common in African American transplant candidates than in whites because they have more possible antigen combinations than whites do, and some of those antigens are very rare in the general population. Scientists are still debating the precise physiology of organ rejection, and particularly the extent to which the organ is jeopardized by less-than-perfect antigen matching.[70] What they do know is that black transplant recipients are more likely to reject their new kidneys. Possible reasons include poor control of hypertension or a more vigorous immune response.[71] Even well-matched transplants can be lost to rejection, suggesting that the standard antigen-matching system may be too simplistic.[72]

Clearly, we need a better understanding of transplant immunology and more effective medicines to prevent rejection.[73] If the compatibility is marginal, it is sometimes most practical for the physician to have the patient stay on dialysis longer to wait for a better match. First, losing a kidney to rejection from mismatch actually makes the recipient more likely to reject future kidneys. Second, every rejected kidney is one less donor kidney that could have been available to another person on the waiting list. This is a critical point because donor kidneys are among the nation's scarcest resources. In 1999, for example, more than 70,000 Americans began dialysis for severe renal disease, but only about 12,500 received transplants.[74]

To circumvent some of the biological constraints, physicians encourage donation of a kidney from a living relative so that the chance of a match will be enhanced. Living donation is also promoted even if the donor is not related and not of the same race because there is so much added benefit from getting a fresh kidney—one that goes straight from the operating room of a healthy donor to the operating room of the recipient without spending too much time on ice. In fact, along with tissue compatibility and the clinical condition of the recipient, the amount of time spent in "cold storage" is one of the most important factors in the successful functioning of a transplanted organ.

Getting a live kidney has little to do with the medical establishment and a great deal to do with the health and attitude of one's family and others of one's own race. Unfortunately, the black donation rate from living individuals is very low relative to need. In 1998, for example, 438 living kidneys were donated by African Americans, but 14,923 African Americans needed a kidney (a ratio of 3 donated per 100 needed), while 2,559 whites gave live kidneys and 20,616 were in need (a ratio of 12 per 100).[75] In addition to personal reluctance and wariness of the system, the low rate of black live donation relative to need is due in part to the fact that so many potential donors are not eligible to give a kidney because they suffer from hypertension or diabetes, conditions that diminish the health of their kidneys.[76] UNOS data show that in 1998 almost one-third of all transplant candidates received a living kidney: 73 percent of those kidneys were given by white individuals to their relatives or friends, and 13 percent by African Americans to theirs.[77]

Most patients on dialysis, especially black individuals, receive an organ from a deceased donor, a so-called cadaveric donor. Once on the waiting list, how do black patients fare in the allocation of kidneys from cadavers? In 1998 African Americans represented 36 percent of the waiting list for kidneys; as a group, they donated 11 percent of all cadaveric kidneys (proportionate to their representation in the general population) and received 27 percent of all donated kidneys.[78]

Thus, more than half of all cadaver kidneys received by black transplant recipients came from donors of other races (predominantly white). As Maritza Rozon-Solomon and Dr. Lewis Burrows of the Department of Surgery at Mount Sinai School of Medicine observe: "African-Americans have historically donated significantly fewer cadaver kidneys than they have received. They have benefitted from Caucasian organ donation."[79]

Donation is a gift of life that transcends racial score-keeping, but it is still important to look closely at the numbers when bias in the allocation of kidneys is alleged.

Cultural Competence

Communication between doctor and patient has always been a vital aspect of the clinical encounter. And with more groups of non-English-speaking immigrants in need of health care, the doctor-patient liaison has taken on added importance. The term "cultural competence" has been coined to refer to the attitudes and activities surrounding such communication. A culturally competent physician, according to the American Medical Association, is one familiar with the "beliefs, values, actions, customs, and unique health needs of distinct population groups."[80]

Cultural competence is really a matter of common sense. Doctors and nurses who serve communities of unacculturated immigrants or isolated rural populations need to learn local anthropology: dietary habits, child-rearing practices, folk remedies, colloquial terms for common symptoms and syndromes, family structure characteristics, attitudes toward physicians and theories of disease causation and prevention. Translators are often needed because it can be awkward and unproductive for a patient's English-speaking child or neighbor to interpret intimate medical details or translate matters like sexual problems, injuries caused by domestic abuse and so on.

Appreciation for these accommodations has grown markedly over the last decade. A recent best-seller about an immigrant Hmong family and its encounter with American medicine is a poignant true story of cultural differences. In *The Spirit Catches You and You Fall Down,* a Hmong daughter is afflicted with epilepsy.[81] The family, attributing her illness to spirits, rebuffs modern medicine. In this account there are no villains. The book, I am told, has become de facto required reading among medical students. The Harborview Medical Center in Seattle and the Metropolitan Health Plan of Hennepin County, Minnesota, have created first-rate interpreter services for their immigrant patients. Other hospitals and health plans have set up community-based interpreter banks that operate in conjunction with local universities and immigrant service agencies. The Kaiser Permanente Medical Center has produced a series of provider handbooks that are packed with technical references, facts on disease patterns, anthropological detail and helpful advice.

Kaiser's seventy-six-page handbook on Asian American and Pacific Island American populations reminds doctors to "ask the patient to whom he or she wants medical information communicated. Among some groups, the patient's hearing of bad news is believed to speed up the process of death."[82] They are also cautioned to "be aware of such practices as coining [rubbing a coin on the body] or cupping to avoid mistaking the reddened areas or marks on the skin as self-abuse or child abuse."[83] From the handbook on Latino populations, clinicians learn that "some Latinas do not breastfeed out of a belief that it is not 'modern' to do so."[84] And "a belief that the life force dwells in the heart is not uncommon and hence such concepts as 'brain death' are less readily understood by some Latinos."[85]

Currently, almost all of the 125 accredited American medical schools offer some teaching in cultural competence. Many add it to their required course on doctor-patient communication, a staple of the first- or second-year curricula when trainees start learning how to interview patients, elicit symptoms and establish rapport. According to the Association of American Medical Colleges, 36 schools had a separate required course on cultural competence in the 1998–99 academic year.[86] Hospitals and health plans are also providing training in cultural competence.

Not surprisingly, some institutions offer variants of cultural competence training. Some programs lapse into a bid for celebrating cultural relativism in the clinical setting, an approach that is not always in the best interest of the patient. The Office of Minority Health of the U.S. Public Health Service, for example, asserts that "culturally competent policies and programs must be developed and implemented in a manner that does not conflict or require change of the beliefs and behaviors of those belonging to a racial or ethnic group being served."[87] Deborah L. Gould, M.D., of the Permanente Medical Group believes that cultural competence requires that a health professional "get past one's own socialization ... [and reexamine] old assumptions regarding the needs and the diagnoses and treatment of patients based upon a predominantly homogeneous Western white model."[88]

Such endorsements of cultural relativism can make it very difficult for doctors to give important advice, according to Dr. Michael Fetters, a Michigan family practice physician. Fetters started the Japanese Family Health Program in Ann Arbor to serve the Japanese families who moved to the area to work for Toyota.[89] His pregnant patients often decline the folate supplements he prescribes to prevent spina bifida and related spinal cord defects, a common prenatal care practice in the United States. In Japan, Fetters explains, vitamins are considered medicine, and medicine is not to be taken during pregnancy. Yet Fetters's patients are not served by a doctor who stands by in the name of cultural sensitivity when unenlightened health practices prevail. The physician must acknowledge the patient's belief, but it is also his ethical imperative to make a tactful attempt to change a patient's mind about taking the supplement. As Fetters says, providing culturally sensitive care doesn't mean you will always meet your patients' expectations.

Wanted: Good Doctors for All Americans

According to a 1994 Harris poll for the Commonwealth Fund, race does not play an especially large role in patients' attitudes about their doctors. When asked to cite the factors that "influence your choice of doctor," the physician's "nationality/race/ethnicity" ranked twelfth out of thirteen possible options.[90] Just 5 percent of whites and 12 percent of minorities said it was important. A greater portion of Asians, 28 percent, rated race/ethnicity as important, probably owing to language barriers.[91] Even so, over 60 percent of white, black and Hispanic respondents said they did not consider the doctor's ability to speak their language particularly relevant to their choice of doctor.[92]

For the entire group of four thousand respondents, factors such as ease of getting an appointment, the convenience of the office location and the doctor's reputation were most influential, cited by about two-thirds of respondents.[93] When respondents who expressed dissatisfaction with their regular doctor were asked for details, only Asians claimed that race or ethnicity was the problem. (And the percentage was small—only 8 percent of all Asian respondents.[94]) Among the subset of the entire sample who said they "did not feel welcome" at their doctor's office, a mere 2 percent of African Americans and Hispanics and 4 percent of Asians attributed the discomfort to racial-ethnic differences.[95]

The main complaint of almost all groups was the doctors' "failure to spend enough time with me."[96] And of those who were dissatisfied enough to change doctors, only 3 percent of Asians and 2 percent of blacks did so on the basis of the physician's race or ethnicity.[97] The most common complaints were "lack of communication," "didn't like him or her," "couldn't diagnose problem" and "didn't trust his or her judgment."[98] Less than 1 percent of those who said they had limited choice about where to get care attributed it to racial or ethnic discrimination.[99]

In focus groups commissioned by the Henry J. Kaiser Family Foundation, discussions revealed that "the most common form of discrimination described by minority consumers was not racial [or] ethnic, rather it was discrimination based on the ability to pay for health services."[100] A 1999 survey by the foundation queried almost thirty-nine hundred people about their doctor. Around 85 percent of whites, African Americans and Latinos rated their doctor as good or excellent.[101] Whites and blacks were about equal in answering "yes" when asked whether their clinician paid enough attention to them (89 and 87 percent, respectively), though slightly fewer Hispanic patients said so (80 percent).[102] One in five black individuals preferred a doctor of their own race, while 12 percent did not want a doctor of their own race.[103] Among Hispanics polled, 28 percent wanted a doctor of their own race, and 17 percent said they did not. In a much smaller survey sponsored by Morehouse College of Medicine in Atlanta, 28 percent of the 251 African Americans surveyed "considered it important that their doctor be of the same ethnic group as themselves."[104]

While most minority patients seem unconcerned about their doctor's race, it is important to some. People with private insurance or enough money can choose their doctor based on race or any other criteria they like, but those in managed care plans are limited to the plan's physician network. The American Association of Health Plans is acutely aware of this. "Plans make a concerted effort to employ a diverse panel of doctors. They want to accommodate patients if they can," I was told by Dr. Charles M. Cutler, chief medical officer of the association.

The data support him. A study of thirteen large urban counties in California conducted by Andrew B. Bindman and his colleagues at the San Francisco General Hospital found that "non-white physicians were no more likely to be denied or terminated from [managed care plans] and HMO contracts than were white physicians."[105] Their sample was representative of the region's physicians, containing more than 70 percent of all office-based black physicians in San Francisco and surrounding areas. A nationwide survey by Elizabeth R. Mackenzie and her colleagues at the University of Pennsylvania also found that a physician's race was not a predictor for whether he would apply to work for a managed care network and his subsequent acceptance.[106]

Nonetheless, the National Medical Association claims that black physicians are being kept from participating in managed care. In January 2000 the association held a press conference to publicize the charge that managed care plans discriminate against them. The group's president, Dr. Walter Shervington, said that "health plans are systematically excluding black physicians from physician panels nationwide. The omission limits patient choice in selecting physicians of like background, ultimately compromising quality health care for the patient and the community."[107] When asked for evidence by a correspondent for *The NewsHour with Jim Lehrer* on PBS, Shervington had none at hand. "Association members conceded that they lacked comprehensive national data to buttress their claims," said the *NewsHour* correspondent.[108]

Indeed, Mackenzie's group found that managed care patients represent a larger proportion (80 percent) of black doctors' practices than of the practices of white doctors (76 percent), Asian doctors (66 percent) and Hispanic doctors (57 percent). Thus, while charges of systematic discrimination are unfounded, the anecdotal reports of black physicians being denied acceptance onto managed care panels no doubt reflect some basic facts about the way managed care, for better or worse, runs its business. For example, managed care plans prefer to hire board-certified physicians (to avert the risk of malpractice), physicians with large practices and those whose patients have private insurance. Relative to white physicians, blacks are less likely to be certified and more likely to be solo practitioners and to treat patients who are under- or uninsured.

Rationale for Affirmative Action in Medical School

Whether the quality of health care for minority patients truly depends on producing greater numbers of minority physicians is an unresolved empirical question. If anything, the evidence we have thus far suggests that the answer is no. Nonetheless, proponents of racial preferences in medical school admissions contend that white physicians treat white patients better than minority patients, with whom, it is said, they have difficulty developing a rapport.[109] "This is not a quota born out of a sense of equity or distribution of justice, but a principle that the best health care may need to be delivered by those that fully understand a cultural tradition," says George Mitchell, the former Senate majority leader and the chairman of the Pew Health Professions Commission.[110]

To be sure, understanding a patient's cultural tradition is important, but need one be a product of that tradition to have sufficient sensitivity to the patient? Virtually all of the major medical organizations, including the AMA and the federal Council on Graduate Medical Education, say yes. Foremost among them is the Association of American Medical Colleges.[111] When California and Texas were planning to dismantle racial preferences in 1996, the AAMC formed Health Professionals for Diversity, a coalition of major medical, health and educational associations, to lobby for the preservation of preferences. By the time Initiative 200, the Washington State referendum to prohibit preferences by race, ethnicity or sex in public institutions, was on the ballot in 1998, the coalition included fifty-one associations among its membership. According to an association vice president, the true message of race-neutral policy to minority students is: "We don't want you."[112]

Given the relatively small numbers of black, Hispanic and Native American physicians (3 percent, 5 percent and less than 1 percent of the nation's medical workforce, respectively), compounded by the declining number of minority applicants in the late 1990s, medical schools know they need to rely on racial preferences if they are to boost these numbers in the next few years.[113] Thus, a few weeks before Washington State voters were to cast ballots on Initiative 200, the AAMC made a highly visible appeal in newspapers. It ran a full-page ad in which eight doctors appear under a huge banner headline: "The Toxic Side-Effects of Initiative 200."

The AAMC's ad warned readers that without racial preferences in medical school admissions, minority Americans will not get the health care they need. After all, the association argued, minority physicians tend to serve black, Hispanic and poor patients more often than white physicians do and are more likely to practice in poor neighborhoods.[114] In addition, the association pointed out, minority medical students often state that they want to practice in medically underserved areas. The ad was also quite specific in predicting that, with fewer minority researchers, less progress will be made in dealing with sickle-cell anemia, prostate cancer and infant mortality—all conditions that disproportionately affect African Americans.

The Current Status of Minorities in Medical Schools

Blacks, Hispanics and Native Americans together represent more than one-fifth of the nation's population but less than one-tenth of the physician workforce. As such, they are underrepresented minorities, or "URMs," as the Association of American Medical Colleges refers to them. Asian Americans are not considered a minority because they are well represented among practicing physicians—10 percent versus 4 percent of the general population—and they represent 18 percent of medical school graduates.[115]

Racial preferences have played a role in raising first-year enrollment to the point where, by 1999, it reached 8 percent black and about 7 percent Hispanic, though it remains 1 percent Native American.[116] But recruitment has been difficult. In 1995, when racial preferences in medical schools were nearly universal, only about 12 percent of first-year students were black, Hispanic or Native American. Robert G. Petersdorf, former president of the AAMC, describes the recruitment challenge: "We cannot produce underrepresented minority medical students if there is an insufficient number who are applying to our schools, graduating from college, or even finishing high school with sufficient skills to enable them to survive a premedical course of study."[117]

Nonetheless, by 2010 the AAMC hopes to attain racial and ethnic representation among physicians that is in proportion to the general population. That goal will be unreachable if current trends continue, according to Donald L. Libby of the Wisconsin Network for Health Policy Research and his colleagues.[118] Based on a minimum requirement of 218 physicians per 100,000 population, Libby calculates that, starting in 1998, the annual number of first-year residents must roughly double for Hispanic and black physicians and triple for Native American physicians if parity is to be attained by 2010. Simultaneously, the number of white first-year residents will have to be reduced by about two-fifths and the number of Asian first-year residents by two-thirds.

The impact of race-neutral policies in some states will make the 2010 parity goal even more elusive. Within two years after Proposition 209 passed in 1996, there was a 29 percent drop in applications by minorities to six public medical schools in California.[119] This set alarm bells ringing throughout the medical establishment. "There is a national health need for physicians who, after the Tuskegee Syphilis Study, for example, are trusted by large segments of our population," wrote Michael J. Scotti Jr. of the American Medical Association. "It would be deplorable," he continued, "if medical schools were not permitted to consider the needs of patients when determining their criteria for selecting the best qualified applicants."[120]

David M. Carlisle and his colleagues at the UCLA School of Medicine proclaimed it a "tragedy that medical students may think they are not welcome . . . within the medical profession."[121] Randall Morgan, an orthopedic surgeon and former president of the National Medical Association (NMA), which represents more than twenty thousand of the nation's African American physicians, said: "War must be declared on any and all attempts to limit access to medical education for students who comprise the under-repre-sented minorities."[122] In protest of the passage of Initiative 200 in Washington, the NMA pulled its 2001 annual meeting from Seattle.[123]

Perhaps the most overwrought statement came from H. Jack Geiger, a professor of public health at the City University of New York. His essay in the *American Journal of Public Health*, "Ethnic Cleansing in the Groves of Academe," foresees these "reversals in minority admissions [as] merely the leading edge of a potential public health disaster."[124] A public health disaster? Only if there is nothing more important to Americans about their doctors than race.

Care Trumps Color

Only a handful of studies have been devoted to the question of whether patients' outcomes are better if they and their doctors are of the same race. Many of these studies were conducted with psychiatric patients, and the majority show that the clinician's race has a minimal impact on how black and white patients fare in their treatment and recovery.[125] One large study that appeared in the journal *Psychiatric Services* involved more than seventeen hundred homeless individuals participating in an intensive services program. Each person was randomly assigned a case manager with whom he worked closely. Over the course of a year improvement in dimensions like the number of days a patient worked at a job, whether he had drug problems and the number of days he spent homeless had no relationship to whether he and the case manager were the same race.[126]

Other researchers looked at the doctor-patient relationship in a different way. One recent study, led by Lisa Cooper-Patrick of the Johns Hopkins University School of Medicine and published in the *Journal of the American Medical Association*, reports that black patients rate their visits as more "participatory" when their doctors are also black.[127] Patients gave the visits a "participation score" based on the frequency with which they felt the doctor involved them in treatment decisions. The Johns Hopkins authors claim that their findings about participation "support the argument for increasing the numbers of minority physicians." Senator Edward M. Kennedy of Massachusetts cited their work as evidence for his assertion that "bias in the health care system is also a factor in racial and ethnic health disparities."[128]

A closer look at the Cooper-Patrick data, however, leaves one unsure about its clinical significance. In particular, patients rated their interactions with a same-race physician (a participation score of 62.6 out of a possible 120) as barely different from interactions with a different-race physician (60.4 out of 120).[129] I questioned Lisa Cooper-Patrick about the clinical significance of such a small numerical difference. She assured me that it was important to the patients' health and referred me to a study by Sherrie H. Kaplan and her colleagues at the New England Medical Center for further confirmation.[130] As it turned out, Kaplan's findings on the relationship of race to the doctor-patient relationship are somewhat different. Her group discovered that minority patients who see minority doctors have *lower* scores on the questions of participation than those who see white doctors.

My point here is not to quibble about conflicting findings by different researchers—this happens routinely in clinical research, especially when the results are not dramatic—but to call attention to a factor that is probably far more important to the doctor-patient relationship than abstract ratings of participation: namely, their time together. Cooper-Patrick found that the duration of a patient's relationship with his physician is linked to higher participatory ratings, comparable to the same-race ratings. Kaplan also found that the amount of time the patient could spend with the doctor helped determine the participation score. In that study, visits of less than twenty minutes appeared to be too brief to involve patients effectively in treatment decisions. Along these lines, another analysis by Kaplan found that physicians who have a "high-volume" practice are rated as less participatory than those who see fewer patients per day.[131]

Thus, in this era of managed care's fifteen-minute doctor visit, what much of the research on attitude really tells us is that most patients attach more value to the amount of time they can spend with their doctor than to the doctor's race or ethnicity. When patients see a different doctor each time they go to the clinic, as is often the case with municipal clinic patients and those whose HMOs have high turnover, it is even harder to establish comfort and trust.

Academic Performance and Racial Preferences

In 1976 Bernard D. Davis, a Harvard microbiologist, found himself at the epicenter of the debate about racial preferences. That year he published an essay in the *New England Journal of Medicine* questioning whether "we have been properly balancing our obligation to promote social justice with our primary obligation to protect the public interest."[132] In his book *Storm over Biology,* Davis elaborated on Harvard Medical School's affirmative action strategy. The medical school dean, Davis said, purposely deprived the medical school faculty of objective feedback on student performance on part of the National Board exam, a test given halfway through medical school: "In the past, the ranking of our students in the National Board Examinations, in each subject, was presented each year at a faculty meeting, and any department that fell below third place in the country virtually apologized. Shortly after the new [minority admissions] program started, the dean's office quietly dropped this annual report."[133]

Eventually, Davis reported, even the National Boards (since replaced by an exam called the United States Medical Licensing Examination) became optional in some cases. He cited the specific example of a minority student who failed the boards *five* times but whom the dean still decided to graduate.

After the publication of his essay, Davis was attacked by the *Harvard Crimson,* picketed by students, roundly criticized by the dean of the medical school and verbally assailed by some of his colleagues. Ultimately, some other colleagues rallied around Davis, pointing out that lowering standards would unfairly put into doubt the qualifications of black and other minorities who would be admitted in the future.

Davis wrote his essay in 1976, but almost twenty-five years later the admissions practices he brought to light still go on in medical schools around the country. Acceptance rates for minority students have long been higher than for white applicants with similar qualifications, according to the Association of American Medical Colleges. In 1979, for example, a minority student with high grades and board scores had a 90 percent chance of being admitted to medical school, while a white applicant with comparable qualifications had a 62 percent chance. By 1991, the last year for which AAMC has published data, the figures were 90 percent versus 75 percent. Conversely, a low-scoring minority applicant had a 30 percent chance of admission while a similarly low-scoring white applicant had a 10 percent chance.

At the University of South Florida College of Medicine, for example, black applicants with a B-plus grade point average (GPA) had a roughly 13 percent chance of admission between 1995 and 1997, but white and Hispanic applicants with the same GPA had only a 4 to 5 percent chance.[134] Despite the passage of Proposition 209 in 1996 in California, minority applicants to some of California's public medical schools were two to almost three times as likely to be admitted as whites and Asians with considerably higher grades.[135]

During the years 1987 through 1993, the medical school of the University of California at San Diego was applying racial preferences. Students accepted through affirmative action had far lower premed course grades and MCAT (Medical College Admissions Test) scores than their fellow white and Asian students. More precisely, the average student accepted through affirmative action had scores comparable to the lowest 1 percent of his white and Asian counterparts. Not among those white students in 1992 was a brilliant computer science major named James Cook. Even though he had graduated Phi Beta Kappa from UC San Diego, he was rejected by its medical school and all the other public California medical schools to which he applied.

Cook's parents were dumbfounded by their son's across-the-board rejection in his home state—especially since he was accepted by the Harvard Medical School. Moved to action, his father obtained copies of the academic records of the students who were admitted to San Diego's medical school over a period of several years. (The race but not the names of the students were made available to Mr. Cook.) With the scatterplots of student scores spread out before him, Cook saw that minority students with lower grades were distinctly favored over white and Asian students with higher grades. In 1994, when he presented the data to a regent of the University of California named Ward Connerly, he touched off the anti–affirmative action campaign that ultimately rocked the state.[136]

Not only are black and Hispanic applicants favored in medical school admissions, but they are overrepresented among students who encounter trouble in medical school. According to the AAMC, they are more likely to repeat their first year or drop out.[137] For the medical school class admitted in 1989, over 20 percent of minority students did not graduate four years later, as is typical. Among white and Asian students, 8 percent did not graduate that year.[138] In 1996 the picture worsened across the board: 39 percent of minority students were unable to keep pace, compared with 15 percent of nonminority students.[139] A 1994 study published in the *Journal of the American Medical Association* found that, in 1988, 51 percent of black medical students had failed part 1 of the National Medical Boards (taken after the second year of medical school), over four times the rate of white students, which was 12 percent. (Failure rates for Hispanic students were 34 percent, and for Asians 16 percent.)[140]

The typical path for students after graduating from medical school is application to a residency program in their chosen specialty. At this level there have also been different outcomes. "It has been documented consistently over the past decade that a higher proportion of underrepresented minority students failed to obtain first-year residency positions through [the standard process]," writes Gang Xu of Jefferson Medical College in Philadelphia and colleagues.[141] Also, the yearly dismissal rate for black residents (14.4 percent) was almost double that for other groups (7.7 percent) from 1996 to 1999.[142] Reasons for dismissal from a residency program can include persistently unprofessional behavior, chronic absenteeism and lack of aptitude or interest.

The problems encountered by black and Hispanic students result from having been underqualified when admitted to medical school. When black students were compared with whites who had similar academic credentials, the failure rates were similar.[143] A 1987 Rand study found that only about one-half of black physicians obtained board certification compared with 80 percent of white physicians. Yet African Americans were *more* likely than white physicians to obtain board certification in a recognized medical specialty if their grades in college and on the Medical College Admissions Test were strong enough to get them admitted on a competitive basis in the first place.[144]

Though the subject deserves more research, a handful of studies have linked medical school performance with the quality of the physician produced. Robyn Tamblyn of McGill University and her colleagues found that licensing examination scores were significant predictors of whether Canadian physicians sought consultations from specialists, prescribed appropriately and ordered screening mammograms for female patients between the ages of fifty and sixty-nine. Given Canada's universal health insurance, these referral and medicating patterns were unlikely to have been influenced by patients' ability to pay.[145] Among American doctors, another study found, having passed the test to become a specialist and the scores received on the internal medical licensing exam were shown to correlate with ratings of performance in practice by fellow doctors.[146]

Students' Needs Versus Patients' Needs

We rely on medical schools to produce qualified pediatricians, surgeons, psychiatrists and other physicians. But admissions preferences violate that trust, despite the schools' good intentions. What would medical schools look like if some of the diversity advocates had their way?

Consider a 1999 essay titled "The Needs of Students from Diverse Cultures," published in *Academic Medicine,* the official, peer-reviewed publication of the Association of American Medical Colleges. The authors, Vera Taylor and George S. Rust of the Morehouse School of Medicine, assert that "many medical schools have difficulty nurturing qualified students from underrepresented minority groups and ensuring that their educational outcomes are comparable to those of non-underrepresented minority students." As they point out:

> In a supportive environment the language levels of textbooks [must be] appropriate to the reading level of the learner. A nursing study

found that [underrepresented minority] students' reading comprehension levels ranged from grades six to 13 while the textbooks' reading levels ranged from grades 12 to 17. The results were a high attrition rate, difficulty in completing the program in four years, and fluctuating pass rates on the Nursing Clinical Licensure Examination. The condition was reversed after faculty and students received training in topics such as reading for the main idea, content mapping, problem solving, and critical thinking. Further studies are needed to determine the extent to which reading issues are a problem in medical education and to identify the most appropriate assessment and remediation tools.

Taylor and Rust also note that minority students are less likely to have a learning style compatible with the lecture format of classroom instruction and that this "may put them at a disadvantage in the first two years of a traditional medical school curriculum."[147]

Should medical and nursing schools be responsible for teaching students to read for the "main idea," something every junior high school graduate should be able to do? To the contrary, teachers who "expect too little" are often cited as a reason that minorities have not enjoyed greater academic advancement and the confidence to pursue medical school.[148]

The authors also worry that minority students "may find the majority institution too individualistic and personally competitive and dissonant with the value they place on cooperation and group success." The American Medical Student Association echoes the concern about the supposed fragility of minority students. "What kinds of psychological preparation and counseling should a person of color have prior to becoming a student at a predominately Caucasian medical school?" the association asks in its publication "Minority Medical Education Assessment Tool and Guidebook," sponsored in part by the federal Bureau of Health Professions.[149]

The guidebook also contains minority medical student complaints. One focus group participant remarks that they encountered "a lack of respect by their colleagues and faculty toward their ambitions to pursue medical careers." It is difficult to know what to make of the complaint about not getting respect, since focus groups that are not randomly selected, like the guidebook's, do not draw a sample that is representative of all miority students. But another problem the students cited is not difficult to interpret: "the inability of elementary and high school systems attended by minority to adequately prepare students for college-level science."

The Intangible Edge

As everyone knows, medical students with strong scores and college (premed) grades do not necessarily make good bedside doctors. Conversely, not all good doctors had brilliant scores and grades in college and medical school. Social skills are very important for a physician, especially a general practitioner. Accordingly, the AAMC has developed a curriculum called the Expanded Minority Admission Exercise to train medical school admissions committees in the use of "non-cognitive variables for the assessment of minority students."[150] It measures seven strengths that are "believed to predict minority students' success": leadership, realistic self-appraisal, determination and motivation, family and community support, social interest, maturity and coping capability and communication skills. The AAMC conducts workshops at various medical schools, using videotapes of sample interviews with minority applicants to demonstrate "interview techniques and culturally sensitive questions."

To be sure, lower grades and scores may not accurately reflect the abilities of some disadvantaged students. But if noncognitive criteria have merit, must they be limited to minority students? Why should some students be judged on grades and test scores and others on more subjective abilities—solely on the basis of race? A more practical question is whether noncognitive variables can predict performance in medical school. While numerous analyses show that MCAT scores are good predictors of clerkship and board performance, almost no studies make a strong case for nonquantitative measures.[151]

Robert C. Davidson and Ernest L. Lewis of the University of California at Davis School of Medicine examined the use of social variables in admissions.[152] The authors analyzed data from 1968 to 1987 on medical students at Davis and compared the academic progress of two groups: regular admissions (of which 4 percent were underrepresented minorities) and "special consideration admissions," which included students granted racial-preference admission as well as nonminority students who appeared to possess the intangible edge bestowed by noncognitive leadership skills. The latter were applicants whose college grades and board scores were less than the recommended minimum but who had other qualities, such as leadership skills, unique life experiences, fluency in languages or "evidence of overcoming barriers such as poverty or physical disability."

In any given year between 10 and 45 percent of all students admitted were special consideration admissions. Students admitted under racial preferences were a large subset of the special consideration admissions—about half during the years examined. The average GPA for the special group was 3.05 (about a B), while regular entrants had a 3.5 (between a B-plus and an A-minus).

As a whole, the applicants who received special consideration fared less well academically than those who were not given special consideration. The authors did not separate out the race-based special consideration entrants; thus, no conclusions could be drawn about racial preferences. The special consideration group had far lower grades in medical school courses and lower scores on parts 1 and 2 of the National Medical Boards. The rates of failure on part 1, which assesses competence in basic sciences such as gross anatomy, pharmacology and pathology, were six times higher among the special consideration students.

Outreach Programs: The Responsible
Road to Diversification

Efforts to increase opportunities for the educationally disadvantaged should start long before students apply to medical school. A strong proponent of early preparation is the former nominee for surgeon general Dr. Henry W. Foster Jr. In a 1994 speech at the AAMC's annual meeting, he noted that "the deficit in performance by underrepresented minorities emanates primarily from being inadequately prepared educationally for the rigor of the premedical curriculum, usually starting in kindergarten and progressing through college. This is, therefore, the current state of the underrepresented minority medical school applicant pool." Foster also noted pointedly that "a few weeks of remedial work prior to entering medical school is insufficient to compensate for years of faulty preparation."[153]

Numerous programs, federal and private, sponsor outreach. The National Institute of General Medical Science at NIH offers grants to colleges and universities to increase the number of underrepresented minorities in biomedical studies. It also sponsors the Bridges to Baccalaureate Degree program for junior college and community college students. The NIH has the Science Education Partnership Awards for K-12 students and Research Supplements for Underrepresented Minorities program for high school and college students.[154] The Bureau of Health Professions of HHS finances yearlong postbaccalaureate programs in fourteen medical schools to prepare minority and disadvantaged students who plan to reapply to medical school after an unsuccessful attempt.

Private organizations such as the Robert Wood Johnson Foundation, the Henry J. Kaiser Family Foundation, the Howard Hughes Medical Institute and the Josiah Macy Jr. Foundation target elementary, high school and undergraduate students and offer scholarships, enhanced science curricula and links to mentors in academic medical centers. The AAMC's Minority Medical Education Program enhances the competitiveness of undergraduates preparing for medical school admission and introduces them to medicine through summer programs at a number of medical schools. To be eligible, a student must be an underrepresented minority and have a minimum overall grade point average of at least 3.0 (B), with at least 2.75 (B-minus) in the sciences. In addition, many university medical centers have begun outreach programs with local colleges and high schools, many through a partnership between the Robert Wood Johnson Foundation and AAMC called the Health Professions Partnership Initiative. These efforts, not lowered standards, are the key to a more diverse workforce.

An Honest Debate

Instituting racial preferences to achieve the goal of diversity for its own sake or in the spirit of compensation for historical mistreatment are philosophical abstractions for debate in courtrooms, classrooms and legislatures. Instituting preferences in order to enhance minority health, however, is a practical proposition that can be tested using real-world data. Thus far, the case has yet to be made that improving minority health depends on having more minority doctors.

It appears that racial preferences represent an inefficient way to increase the number of minority doctors—and thus minority health—for several reasons. First, minority representation in medical schools remains well below their representation in the general population, despite aggressive admissions policies.[155] Second, minority recruitment has resulted in a two-tiered system of academic standards for admission. This has created attendant problems: some potential nonminority medical students have not been treated fairly, while some minority students have embarked upon a career for which they are ill prepared. Third, we lack compelling evidence that same-race (minority) doctor-patient relationships result in better patient outcomes.

No matter who treats our nation's poor and minority patients, the fact is that they tend to have multiple, chronic medical conditions and are often clinically complicated. They need the best doctors they can get, regardless of race. Fortunately, inner-city poor and minority patients are most likely to get their care in high-volume municipal hospitals that are associated with academic medical centers and thus have better access to resources and technical support. They employ experienced physicians who perform hundreds of the same operations each year.[156] Over half of all patients hospitalized in major teaching hospitals in 1995 were uninsured, poor or minority, a Rand evaluation found. Black and poor patients received *better* care in urban teaching hospitals than white and more affluent patients received in rural or nonteaching urban hospitals.[157]

But ambulatory care is a different story. There are not enough doctors choosing to work in rural community clinics and poor, inner-city neighborhoods. In a numbem of states, such as Florida, Illinois, North Dakota, Texas and New York, graduates of foreign medical schools represent one-fourth to one-half of the physician workforce in underserved areas.[158] California has approved legislation requiring its public medical schools to increase the number of training slots for primary care physicians and decrease slots for specialists.[159] Some rural and inner-city communities have used creative financial incentives (for example, loan forgiveness, rent rebates, higher pay) to draw young doctors to their area. We should be promoting such strategies, not lowering standards for admission to medical school.[160] As far as patient preferences are concerned, again, it makes more sense to create mechanisms of health care coverage that ensure patient choice than to open the doors of medical schools to unprepared students.

Finally, we must not forget that the physician is part of a larger network of health care providers. For some preventive care (such as vaccinations for children and the elderly, prenatal care, routine baby checkups and blood pressure surveillance), physicians are not even needed. Specially trained nurses can help provide after-hours medical appointments and give basic advice over the telephone. Public health nurses or physician assistants cooperating with local churches and community organizations can deliver these services at least as effectively. Inner-city hospitals are now hiring health educators (ideally from within the community) to teach fellow residents about diet and exercise, smoking cessation and screening for cancer, diabetes and hypertension. These workers also participate in outreach to get people into clinics for routine care, efforts that are so important because medically indigent people tend to underuse available care, to show up in emergency rooms for minor problems and to delay seeking diagnoses for conditions like cancer until an advanced stage.

While well-meaning groups like the AAMC advance the questionable belief that minority health is dependent on minority physicians, experience points toward the virtue of expending energy and resources on the solutions outlined in chapter 1 if we are to narrow the health gap. These include promoting health literacy, forming community health organization partnerships and expanding health coverage to the uninsured. What patients seem to want most is a qualified doctor who will spend unhurried time with them. The racial disparities in health are real, but data do not point convincingly to systematic racial bias as a determinant. Nor does the evidence suggest that racial preferences in medical school admissions are the remedy for health disparities.

7

Therapy for Victims

WHEN MELODIE J. PEET was commissioner of mental retardation and substance abuse services for the state of Maine, from 1994 to the summer of 1999, she made it a priority to develop treatment services for women who, like herself, had been mistreated as children. Soon after Peet settled into her job, she told a gathering of mental health professionals: "I haven't seen or heard anything that leads me to believe that a trauma survivor in Maine today can walk into any treatment facility . . . and be sure that she is going to be treated seriously."[1] And there are a lot of survivors. Maine's Office of Trauma Services estimates that 95 percent of the women who use the department's services were abused in childhood.[2]

Melding antipsychiatry animus with the feminist-inspired "trauma" movement, Peet established an Office of Trauma Services within her agency. Chosen to head the Office of Trauma Services was Ann Jennings, who also had personal ties to the trauma movement. Her daughter Anna was sexually abused by a baby-sitter during the years when Jennings herself had a severe drinking problem. At age thirty-two, Anna hanged herself in a California state mental hospital. Jennings now lectures and writes about Anna's experiences; she even wrote her doctoral dissertation on Anna's ordeal, blaming the mental health system for her daughter's death since it failed to recognize that her problems sprang from her sexual violation in childhood.

No one would dare dispute that Anna, as a child, had been a victim or that her death was a tragedy for her mother. But I seriously question whether having access to "trauma services," with their relentless harping on victimhood, would have saved Anna's young life. Nevertheless, the trauma services movement—based on the premise that early trauma inevitably produces catastrophic problems needing special treatment—is gaining momentum.

As the 1990s wound down, Florida, Massachusetts, New Hampshire, Ohio, Rhode Island, Texas, Wisconsin and Wyoming were all considering establishing a trauma office in their department of mental health. In 1999 the federal Substance Abuse and Mental Health Services Administration made $40 million in grants available to applicants who wanted to develop trauma programs for women. The National Association of State Mental Health Program Directors approves of this trend: "Psychological effects of violence and trauma in our society are pervasive, highly disabling yet largely ignored. [We] believe that responding to behavioral health care needs of men, women and children who have experienced trauma should be a priority of state mental health programs."[3]

The trauma movement crystallized in the late 1980s with the publication of the best-selling *The Courage to Heal.* The book fueled the false (repressed) memory craze by informing its readers, "If you think you were abused and your life shows the symptoms, then you were."[4] Pop psychologists are not the only ones who have sought to legitimize so-called repressed memories of abuse. At the scholarly end of the feminist spectrum is the Harvard psychiatrist Judith Lewis Herman, who insists that "the ordinary response to atrocities is to banish them from consciousness."[5] Remembering, she says, is a prerequisite for healing. But is it? What is the evidence? At bottom, of course, child abuse does happen. But for unknown reasons, only some people are left with gaping psychic wounds. At stake ultimately is the issue of how those who have been so staggeringly betrayed by trusted adults can go on to lead productive, untormented lives. Children are certainly not responsible for their maltreatment at the hands of adults, but when they grow up they are accountable for the present and must strive to determine their future. Trauma-sensitive treatment, as we will see, threatens to keep them mired in the past.

This chapter has three interwoven sections. First, I focus on Maine as a case study in the development of trauma-sensitive services because it is further along than other states in establishing these services. As we will see, Maine has not based its innovation on sound clinical principles. For example, there is no solid scientific base to support the twin assumptions that recollections of trauma are inevitably accurate and, more important, that focusing on them is necessarily beneficial. Like the consumer-survivors in Chapter 2, proponents of the Maine plan challenge the expertise of professionals. Further, the Maine philosophy holds that trauma patients, mostly women, have been made sick by the brutality of fathers and brothers—in other words, by men. Writes Judith Herman: "The study of trauma . . . becomes legitimate only in a context that challenges the subordination of women and children."[6]

This last notion—of being made mentally ill by an oppressor—links the story of Maine with the other two parts of this chapter. The latter sections explore feminist psychotherapy and multicultural counseling, what I call oppression-based therapies. The "oppression therapists" bring their politics to the couch, telling patients that psychological troubles arise from living in a sexist or racist society and even encouraging them to become politically active. Sadly, it is the therapists themselves, despite their good intentions, who may be the victimizers.

Precursors of Maine's Victim-Oriented Approach

Traditionally, distress related to childhood trauma has been considered one among many adult mental conditions. Patients who were abused as children were treated on inpatient wards or in clinics along with everyone else with a mental problem or illness. Asking about aspects of a patient's childhood—ideally in a nonleading, open-ended manner—was a standard part of the interviewing procedure. The clinician, for example, might ask the patient, "When you were growing up, was there ever any behavior in your family that you considered—at the time or now, in retrospect—abusive or sexually inappropriate?" But in recent years many therapists have come to insist that adults who were victimized in childhood require specialized treatment.

An early model for trauma-based treatment arose in the mid-1980s in the form of specialized wards in psychiatric hospitals. These were often run by all-female staff and usually treated only women. Sometimes staff were expressly hostile to male psychiatrists; a number of my male colleagues have told me they were asked to leave if they entered the trauma ward—to conduct administrative business with the head nurse, for example—because the staff feared their presence would "upset the women."

In the era before managed care, patients used to remain in the hospital for about a month in places like the Sanctuary, a private inpatient trauma program near Philadelphia. Sandra Bloom, the psychiatrist who developed the Sanctuary, wrote a book called *Creating Sanctuary* in which she endorses the importance of remembering and then reliving long-repressed traumas. Memories of traumatic experiences, she writes, "must be assumed to have at least some basis in reality."[7] Unfortunately, her assumptions are flawed.

First, a therapist cannot automatically assume that formerly "banished" memories of child abuse are true. Second, if true, it is not necessarily the case that they are at the root of a person's current symptoms and life circumstances. Adults who are depressed or unfulfilled, for example, often attribute their current misery to prior stressful events, magnifying their importance in retrospect. Also, formative (or deformative) experiences are vastly complex. Child abuse takes place in a developmental context that generally includes other forms of maltreatment and degrees of family dysfunction, disruption and deprivation.[8] Conversely, many people who experienced severe early trauma have no measurable psychopathology as adults.[9]

Good data about the incidence of child abuse and the effectiveness of treatments are hard to come by. Asking adults about childhood experiences can produce reports that are false or grossly exaggerated; on the other hand, the researcher who relies on self-reports can also miss cases. Few researchers have even attempted to procure documenting evidence. In addition, most studies are cross-sectional; ideally, researchers would perform follow-up analyses to determine whether children who have endured actual events grow up to develop problems. Granted, this kind of research is enormously time-consuming, but it is needed. Without it, we know little about the scope of the problem and cannot discern which innovations are worth replicating on a larger therapeutic scale.

The notion that it is beneficial to dwell on early trauma rests on similarly shaky ground. Many people who talk about their traumatic experiences do no better than those who are more stoic about their pain.[10] Sometimes, in fact, they feel more depressed and function at a lower level than their less emotive counterparts when evaluated over time. The same dynamic has been observed in patients recovering from heart attacks and in war veterans, Holocaust survivors and bereaved spouses.[11] Moreover, traumatized people who talk relentlessly about their anguish often end up driving away friends and loved ones, the very people who form their support network.[12]

The treatment of adults with childhood trauma is also a poorly researched area. Most informative are analyses of interventions with newly traumatized adults. Studies of rape victims reveal that after a five-week program in which the women were told to reexperience the rape, the majority no longer had nightmares and other symptoms compared to rape victims who underwent supportive counseling.[13] Even here, however, not all of the patients benefited, underscoring the fact that there is no one-size-fits-all method of coping with trauma.

Sandra Bloom offers no data about treatment success at the Sanctuary. Nonetheless, she is optimistic that "some of the insights we have gained from our work with some of the most injured warriors in the battle of life can contribute to an interdisciplinary, interracial, transgendered, global conversation leading to a new, more humane and attainable vision for the centuries to come."[14]

Though she may wax grandiose in places, one cannot read Bloom's book and doubt that she is sincerely concerned for patients and for social justice. But good intentions are not enough to keep some patients from burrowing deeper into themselves, especially when they are encouraged, relentlessly, to focus on traumatic experiences. My colleague Dr. G told me about such a patient, Valerie W. While he was making daily rounds in a big-city emergency room, he was called to see Valerie, a woman in her mid-twenties. He entered the room to find a large woman, perhaps five-feet-ten, in a fetal position on a gurney, clutching a teddy bear whose name was "Strength." At the foot of the gurney were two large shopping bags that contained her worldly possessions.

Valerie told Dr. G her story while still huddled in the fetal position. She had experienced years of depression, stormy and unsatisfactory relationships and preoccupation with ideas of suicide. Valerie attributed her symptoms to the fact that she had been sexually abused by her father over a period of several years while a teenager. She exhibited "no need for recovered memories," Dr. G said to me, because "she had never forgotten." Despite her distress, which was considerable, she had attended and finished a two-year college and had a reasonably good job, an apartment, and a car. Then, six months before, she had found a new therapist after a disagreement with her old one. The new therapist made the sexual abuse and the criminal culpability of her father the central focus of their sessions. As the therapy progressed, Valerie told Dr. G, the abuse came to dominate her thoughts. She became more depressed and thought about suicide constantly.

Valerie eventually had to be hospitalized and spent several weeks on a special inpatient unit that focused on abuse. And focus she did. After discharge, Dr. G recalled, she found herself no longer able to work, too absorbed in her memories and too depressed to do much else. Valerie described persistent, intrusive thoughts about the prior abuse that seemed to preclude any ability to focus on the "here and now." She was unable to make payments on her car, which was repossessed, and she had just been evicted from her apartment—the precipitant for the ER visit.

The practical difficulties of getting her appropriate care were formidable. As it was, she would get just a day or so of observation in the hospital, a new script for antidepressants and help finding both a new therapist and a shelter to go to. But Dr. G was even more dismayed by the trampling of Valerie's fragile defenses by her prior therapist and the inpatient unit. "The truth did not set her free," Dr. G remarked, "at least not when delivered by fire hose to a person who was barely holding it together." Dr. G wondered whether the therapist, who was unreachable when he called from the emergency room, considered the treatment a success.

Does the story of Valerie W, a classic case of regression, mean that all patients are harmed by places like the Sanctuary? No. In fact, with short stays of one to two weeks, thanks to managed care, there is probably just enough time for stabilization and respite but not enough for regression. As public mental health systems like Maine's, however, import the dubious tactics of the private "sanctuaries," such casualties may become more frequent.

Maine's Survivors

When Melodie Peet took the reins as mental health commissioner, one of her first acts was to appoint several trauma advisory groups (TAGs) to get a "diverse set of opinions about what facilitates or hinders healing." The TAGs were composed of 127 trauma survivors who had received public mental health services and 122 professionals recommended by those survivors. Participants' comments were published in a 1997 report, *In Their Own Words: Trauma Survivors and Professionals They Trust Tell What Hurts, What Helps and What Is Needed for Trauma Services.*[15]

The report describes itself as representing the "official 'coming out' of those in Maine who have wrestled in frustrated isolation with their own, a loved one's, or a client's history of sexual and physical abuse." At the TAGs, many survivors say that therapists should always ask about past trauma. As one remarks, "Never being asked [by professionals] about trauma is like the abuse as a child. . . . The stigma and silencing of sexual abuse by providers and by society is very hurtful." A number of survivors recommend that they be "brought in [to] tell the psychiatrists and veteran psychiatric nurses and social workers how they have hurt us, why certain standard procedures humiliate, shame, and traumatize us, and how they can work with us to make it better." Another bit of advice from the TAG participants is to "blur the boundaries between consumer/survivors and professionals, soften and break down the barriers." The survivors also have the impression that a high percentage of mental health professionals were themselves trauma survivors who also need treatment because "professionals who haven't dealt with their own abuse can't be helpful."[16]

What do these perceptions and recommendations amount to? Is it necessarily wise to take the advice of needy individuals who themselves seem so confused about reconciling their dependence on therapists with their rejection of patienthood? Bear in mind as well that the TAG participants were not chosen at random. These survivors volunteered for the opportunity to express their dissatisfaction with the system and to suggest improvements; thus it was virtually ensured that the report would reflect the views of a self-selected group of disgruntled individuals (accompanied by therapists of whom they approved) rather than a representative sample of those being treated in the system.

Nevertheless, the TAG event became a stimulus for Peet to organize conferences teaching Maine therapists about the ways in which they had hurt patients and how they could now help them. I attended the second such conference in Portland in October 1998. Most of the roughly five hundred attendees were women. Upon entering the meeting area at the local Holiday Inn, I immediately noticed signs asking participants to "please put beepers on vibrate since some participants have difficulty with the beep sound." A conference coordinator explained that the beeping noise was like the sound of a doctor's beeper or an IV machine—"you know, something that reminds them of a bad experience they had in a hospital."

Other signs posted every thirty feet or so announced the availability and location of two "safe rooms," hotel rooms set aside for participants who felt overwhelmed by anxiety or emotion during the conference. Volunteer safe-room attendants provided emotional support, and the rooms were stocked with art supplies, pens, pencils and paper for self-expression. Unfortunately, the safe rooms didn't provide quite enough safety for one of the participants, who cut her wrists while surrounded by "supporters." I couldn't help but wonder whether this gesture was an act of exhibitionism inadvertently invited by the conference coordinators, who did such a good job of letting the attendees know just how fragile everyone thought they were.

Nancy Coyne, a psychiatrist from Brunswick, Maine, led a session called "Trauma Treatment in the Nineties." The conference program's description of the session was decidedly New Age: "This [seminar] will explore the range of tools available to catalyze and assist the healing process.

Many modes will be addressed: medications, body work, energy work, wilderness experience, art and music, yoga and meditation, journaling/ writing, etc."

"Bodywork" is based on the premise that "the brain/nervous system can only reproduce what it has experienced," explained Karin Spitfire, a counselor from Belfast, Maine. Bodywork practitioners believe that the imprint of physical trauma is manifested in specific bodily sensations (such as pelvic, oral or anal pain), in one's posture or in muscle tension. As Chrystine Oksana theorizes in her book *Safe Passage to Healing: A Guide for Survivors of Ritual Abuse:* "There appears to be both memory and intelligence at the cellular level. . . . The information coming from our bodies is irrefutable. If your body has retained unresolved pain, has scars, or re-enacts an event, you can be sure that the pain, the injury, or the event happened."[17]

Paradoxically, bodyworkers embrace at least one aspect of Freudian theory that Freud himself abandoned as damaging to patients: the theory that daily neuroses are traceable to discrete traumatic events that are not remembered. True, horrific events are sometimes repressed, though this is not common. My own tendency, incidentally, is to believe most patients who have "always" remembered they were mistreated, and to doubt most of those who recently became aware of long-forgotten memories of abuse.

The American Psychological Association is so concerned about the ethical and legal implications of "implanting" memories of abuse through suggestion that it published a primer for therapists called *Treating Patients with Memories of Abuse: Legal Risk Management.* The therapists of Maine, it turns out, violated much of the advice offered by the APA, including this bit of legal wisdom: "Techniques commonly associated with allegations of implanted memories include . . . body work, trance writing, guided imagery, journaling, and dream interpretation."[18] The Maine survivors said these techniques helped them remember abuse from their earliest infancy. Indeed, it was widely accepted by the meeting participants that individuals possess the ability to recall trauma experienced in infancy, notwithstanding the evidence from cognitive science, which indicates that events experienced before the age of two, and perhaps even later, are not retained in recallable memory.

Another session was devoted to lurid descriptions of self-mutilation by women who routinely "self-injured" when they were upset. One member of the audience referred us to a self-help web site she had consulted. It offers the following advice:

> Deciding to stop self-injury (SI) is a very personal decision. You may have to consider it for a long time before you decide you are ready to commit to a life without scars and bruises. Don't be discouraged if you conclude that the time isn't right for you to stop yet . . . you should take care to remain safe when harming yourself: don't share cutting implements and know basic first aid for treating your injuries . . . keep cuts shallow, do only the minimum required to ease your distress. Decide how many cuts, burns, bruises you are going to inflict, decide how deep/severe, how long you will allow yourself to engage in SI.[19]

Cutters, as they are sometimes called, can share their thoughts through an online bulletin board that is sponsored by a group called Bodies Under Siege.[20] Thus, pathology becomes an activity around which to form an identity ("self-injurer") and a social network. The problem with this kind of social network is that the price of belonging is self-harm.

Self-mutilation is often associated with a group of psychiatric patients known as borderlines. The term refers to individuals who sit on the diagnostic border between psychotic and neurotic. Many of the women at the conference said they suffered from a condition called borderline personality disorder (BPD). Distressingly, so did many of the therapists—by their own acknowledgment.

Borderline personality disorder is a condition marked by volatile relationships, poor impulse control and enormous swings in self-regard, from grandiosity to self-loathing. Other symptoms include chronic emptiness and boredom, intense fear of rejection or abandonment and seismic outbursts of rage. Half-hearted, attention-getting suicide attempts are common. People who enter relationships with borderlines describe being whipsawed between feeling desperately needed one moment and hatefully rejected the next. In the notorious "black-and-white" world of the borderline, friends who are idolized one day are degraded the next. Borderlines are famous for the "mixed messages" they broadcast. As we will see, the push-pull nature of borderline pathology meshes nicely with the consumer-survivors' plan for revising Maine's mental health system.

The Cult of the Borderline

The borderlines of Maine want to be competent therapists and needy patients at the same time. They want therapists to listen, but if therapists don't give the correct response, they are called insensitive or, worse, accused of being out to silence survivors. Maine's consumer-survivors don't think they should be blamed if they are difficult to deal with because, after all, the system has retraumatized them. They don't want to be regarded as fragile and unable to make good decisions, yet they will have the unwitting therapist walk on eggshells lest she trigger a mood swing or even a total personality switch. The Maine patients don't want to be "psychiatrically labeled," but they do want to be recognized, accommodated and given disability payments or jobs as peer counselors.

Peet and her colleagues essentially colluded with their confused patients by allowing them to define the terms of their therapy. What these patients needed instead were professionals who encourage accountability and define limits. In short, Peet and company have fashioned a system that looks very much as if it were designed by borderlines for borderlines—a prescription for disaster.

Borderline patients are among the most difficult to treat. Experienced therapists generally limit the number of borderlines in their practice because treating them is so time-consuming and emotionally draining. These patients need solid, well-trained clinicians, but in Maine they are instead seeing low-paid therapists, many of whom have no more than a bachelor's degree. Maine's credentialing process is among the most relaxed in the country. "Almost anyone can hang out a shingle," says Linda Breslin, the retired superintendent of the Augusta Mental Health Institute.

"The therapists of trauma victims are good-hearted but have no scientific grounding and are poorly supervised. I really worry about these patients; they are at severe risk for being maltreated."[21]

Theory and clinical observation suggest that the person with borderline personality disorder has sustained a number of major developmental insults and that these have led to deficiencies in the most basic tasks of living. One is the inability to self-soothe. Most people can tolerate painful emotional states—sadness, disappointment, anger, loss—by telling themselves they'll get through it, by thinking back on other storms they have weathered or by figuring out how to distract themselves in neutral or productive ways. The borderline cannot. A borderline patient may cling to someone she idolizes as her savior only to revile him when he (inevitably) disappoints. Lynn Williams, a woman who says she had "world-class symptoms of BPD," describes herself as follows: "[It is like] having been born without an emotional skin—with no barrier to ward off real and perceived emotional assaults. What would be a headache in emotional terms for someone else was a brain tumor for me. This reaction was spontaneous and not something that I chose. . . . Feelings swept over me like one of those nets used to trap animals in the jungle—black, dark, persistent, and, at times, suicidal feelings. Those feelings, accompanied by flawed logic, fantasies of rescue . . . created chaos in my mind."[22]

The chaos can lead to frightening experiences. When overwhelmed by stress, the borderline may feel numb, as if she does not even exist. This may drive her to mutilate herself. "I felt as if I was isolated from the world, dead, with no emotions at all," a self-abusing woman named Lindsay told Marilee Strong, author of *A Bright Red Scream.* "The blood told me I was alive, that I could feel. I needed to see those bad feelings bleed away. Also I couldn't cry; bleeding was a different form of crying."[23] Other patients burn themselves with lit cigarettes or score their bodies with razor blades or fingernails. Self-mutilation typically begins as an impulsive act but may become ritualized over time.

In addition to alleviating borderlines' misery, effective treatment for people with the disorder would reduce the high social costs of the condition incurred through drug and alcohol abuse, AIDS and other commu-

nicable diseases, gambling, domestic violence, teen pregnancies, run-
aways, overuse of the courts and revolving-door emergency room visits
and hospital stays. Fortunately, there is a promising approach called dialectical behavioral therapy. Developed in 1991 by Marsha Linehan, a
University of Washington psychologist, dialectical therapy has earned the
welcome distinction of having been rigorously tested in clinical trials.[24]

It consists of weekly fifty-minute individual therapy sessions and
two half-hour group therapy sessions per week. The individual session is
devoted to the objective dissection of a particularly difficult event from
the past week. Ancient traumas are not discussed, and memories are not
actively retrieved. In painstaking detail, the patient and the therapist perform a kind of behavioral postmortem, going over the chain of events
leading up to the episode (for example, the patient's angry confrontation
with her spouse or her rejection for a job), reviewing various strategies for
dealing with conflict, and examining the reasons the patient felt unable to
employ those strategies.

The virtues of dialectical therapy underscore the hazards of the
Maine approach. Whereas the dialectical approach helps patients define
boundaries between themselves and others, the Maine therapists encourage dependent attachments, unlimited contact and, in some cases, even
physical touching by the therapist (a thoroughly unacceptable act in conventional psychological treatment). Whereas the dialectical approach in-
stills impulse control and responsibility for soothing one's self, Maine's
infantilizing therapists rush in to gratify. And whereas the dialectical approach tries to solidify a patient's sense of independent self, the Maine
therapists talk of multiple personalities and encourage patients to become
swallowed up in group identity.

Multiple Personality Disorder:
The Perils of Suggestion

A great deal of evidence demonstrates the power of suggestion in shaping
people's memories. Elizabeth Loftus, a University of Washington psychologist, has done numerous studies in which she is able to "create" memo-

ries in college-age volunteers. In one experiment Loftus had subjects view a videotape of an automobile accident and then asked them, "How fast was that car going when it ran the stop sign?" and "How fast was it going when it passed the barn?" Few of the subjects noticed that the film contained neither a stop sign nor a barn.

Suggestibility also plays a role in another phenomenon popular with Maine therapists: multiple personality disorder. A person who has been diagnosed with multiple personality disorder possesses an ideal device for evading accountability and for manipulating others. Being a so-called multiple gives the patient permission to blame her actions on an alternate personality or to conveniently "forget" them. Trauma therapy teaches patients to be wary of "triggers," events that will cause them to switch to another personality. It often backfires, as one therapist told me: "These patients hold the hospital staff hostage by saying, 'If you do that, you are going to trigger me, and then who knows what I'll do?' They know it ties us in knots; we don't want to stress them unduly, but we don't want to be tricked into not holding them responsible."

How common is multiple personality disorder? The *Diagnostic and Statistical Manual of Mental Disorders* (*DSM*) says that about 1 percent of the general population is afflicted, but many psychiatrists think that rate, comparable to the prevalence of schizophrenia, is too high. In the 1980s, at the height of the multiple personality craze, "most psychiatrists had probably still never met a patient with the diagnosis," wrote the psychiatrist Peter D. Kramer.[25] Even the infamous "Sybil," subject of the 1974 best-seller, may have been little more than a profoundly unhappy and suggestible woman. Indeed, Paul McHugh, chairman of the Johns Hopkins University Department of Psychiatry, is skeptical that the personality condition exists at all except as an artifact of the therapist's suggestion. His advice: "Close down the services [designed to treat it] and disperse the patients to general psychiatric units. Ignore the alters. Stop taking notes on them."[26]

Multiple personality disorder can certainly *seem* to manifest itself when the right incentives are present. "The answer to how much of a multiple personality problem there is has to do with the kind of gratification it brings," explains William Anderson, a psychiatrist at Massachusetts General Hospital.[27] "When a person is told that she is one of a special class of patient, given sympathy and therapy sessions and not really expected to act responsibly, you'd be surprised how many patients with multiple personalities there can be on a ward or in a clinic."

When childhood abuse has occurred, a good therapist will help the patient use that experience as one explanation among several for her current state, rather than as a justification for destructive behavior. "The biggest problem [with Maine's approach] is that patients are seduced by the emphasis on trauma," says Dennis Ratner, a psychologist in private practice in Waterville, Maine.[28] Ratner points out that the patients are made to feel that there is something special about being a victim of child abuse. "It has been turned into a cause célèbre by well-meaning but overzealous therapists and administrators and patients who embrace the identity of survivor," he says. A history of sexual abuse becomes the currency in this system, explaining unhappiness and getting attention.

I must point out here that suggestion works in either direction. A therapist who tells a patient that her memories of abuse are unreliable can be just as powerful a figure and as damaging an influence as one who tells her that recollections will return if she just remembers hard enough. I suspect that a large fraction of the female patients in my drug treatment clinic probably did experience some forms of sexual violation as children. Only a handful of them mention this when I first meet them, though many more relate the experience during subsequent visits.

My strategy is to acknowledge the patient's painful past and its unfairness, but to emphasize the here and now. I focus on accepting responsibility for current behavior regardless of the past. If the woman is in a destructive relationship, getting out of it (temporarily or permanently) is generally what our sessions are about. After all, how can she be a responsible mother if she exposes her children to such chaos, disrespect and, often, danger? How can she expect to stay sober if she opens herself up to such misery? In my experience, patients typically concede these truths, and most of them actually follow through on our step-by-step strategy. If a woman wants to talk about "why I get myself into these situations," we can do that. But first, I help her get herself out.

Maine's system takes another approach entirely. In short, it has come to resemble a cult. "Their worldview is that you are either a victim, a perpetrator or a rescuer," Anderson tells me. Critics, of course, are cast in the role of perpetrator by state officials and therapists alike. In the borderline's black-and-white world, evil is personified by the outside universe, and good comes only from within the group. Because borderlines yearn for direction and acceptance, they may be attracted to strong leaders like Peet, Anderson says. The role of survivor is indeed enticing, for it provides instant and unconditional acceptance, automatic intimacy and a paternalistic leader who will be readily idealized.

Breaking away from this fellowship would be difficult for anybody, but it is nearly impossible for someone who derives self-definition and companionship from it and who is terrified of abandonment. According to Roger Wilson, a psychiatrist who has run an inpatient unit at the Bangor Mental Health Institute for twenty years, "It is damaging to patients to focus on their victimhood instead of their strength."[29] Wilson describes a patient he has known since the 1980s. For a while the patient was doing rather well, holding down a job and living independently. "Then, around 1990, when Bangor therapists got into the multiple personality disorder craze, she got involved and regressed tragically," he says. Subsequently, Wilson recalls, the patient has been "hospitalized many times and refuses to leave because she now can't trust her 'alters' not to hurt her."

The Rise of Oppression-Based Therapies

Psychotherapists continue to take the "victim-sensitive" approach into new territory with two new types of therapy—feminist therapy and multicultural counseling, which are flourishing in public and university mental health clinics and enjoy a secure niche in graduate-level training programs. Multicultural counselors populate high schools and social service agencies. Both therapies typify the postmodern approach, assuming that the most important characteristic of a patient is her membership in an oppressed group, and that her psychological distress is a product of conflict between the individual and the sexist and racist society in which the patient lives.

Feminist therapy and contemporary multicultural counseling have their ideological roots in a discipline called community mental health. Community psychologists, in the words of the psychologist Dennis R. Fox, "have long insisted that prevention of mental disorder must begin with widespread and expansive social reform in order to prevent the emotional distress and mental disturbance in our society that is due to dehumanizing social influences such as oppression, meaningless work, racism and sexism."[30]

Feminist psychotherapy reflects this doctrine. According to Laura S. Brown, a prominent "feminist practitioner," psychologist and author of *Subversive Dialogues: Theory in Feminist Therapy,* feminist therapy is "one aspect of the feminist revolution." The therapy functions, writes Brown, "to subvert patriarchal dominance at the most subtle and powerful levels, as it is internalized and personified in the lives of [patients.]"[31] In the dystopic realm of feminist therapy, there seem to be only victims and perpetrators.

In Brown's scheme, society is dysfunctional, not the patient. And because a woman's mental state is believed to reflect the position of women in society, any symptoms of depression or anxiety are seen largely as the product of a society that is hostile to women. Thus, a feminist therapist is often reluctant to suggest to a woman that she might bear some responsibility for her problems at home, in her relationships or with her self-image. Such suggestions risk oppression of the patient by the therapist. The therapist's "power to name and define reality serves to deepen and exacerbate the power imbalance and inequities between the therapist and the client," Brown writes. "This act establishes the authority and expertise of the therapist in no uncertain terms."[32] Well, yes. A patient turns to a therapist for help precisely because he *has* the expertise to take a patient on a guided exploration of the self—the true task of psychotherapy.

But that avenue of exploration is foreclosed when sources of discomfort are so readily identified as external and imposed by a male-dominated society. Consider the way this feminist therapist introduced herself to a new patient, Ruth:

THERAPIST: I bring a social and political perspective to my understanding of you and your life. I believe the causes of the problems many women bring to counseling are external. In general women are not valued by our society and this creates psychological distress.[33]

What follows is a compressed excerpt from a session between this therapist and patient as it appears in *Case Approach to Counseling and Psychotherapy*:

RUTH: I know it sounds silly, but I just feel fat, old and ugly these days.

THERAPIST: But that's the way we are trained to think. And if a woman looks like hell, she feels like hell because she is devalued in our society. . . . Our bodies are the single most powerful asset we have in our society. You might try thinking about your weight by discovering ways in which being fat affords you power in your relationships and begin to love yourself just the way you are.

RUTH: That won't be easy.

THERAPIST: I know. It wasn't easy for me either. . . . I forced myself to look at my body and learn to love it.[34]

In this snippet we see the therapist unduly influencing Ruth. The issue may seem mundane (body image), but no matter what the patient brings to the therapist, the goal should be helping her determine, for herself, how her best interests can be served. Because our feminist therapist happens to resent the notion that some bodies are considered more acceptable than others, she encourages her patient to ignore convention. She assumes that wanting a slim or shapely figure is really about pleasing men and so tells her patient to "love" her body. To the feminist therapist, Ruth's dismay about her body *must* be a product of conflict with "gender-role expectation"—that is, thinness. While there's nothing wrong with loving one's overweight body, a patient should do so because it makes sense to her, not to her therapist.

Feminist therapists also fret about the "power differential" in the therapist-patient relationship. To neutralize this differential, the therapist actively discloses personal details about herself—an unheard-of technique in traditional therapy, which maintains boundaries between doctor and patient in order to preserve the former's objectivity. Some have even struggled with whether to accept payment for their services, since doing so, they fear, enforces the notion of hierarchy.

The feminist therapist is also an activist. "We are aware of the limitations that racism, sexism, classism, anti-Semitism, ageism, heterosexism, ablebodiedism and other oppressions impose on groups and individuals," reads a statement of the Feminist Therapy Institute in Portland, Oregon.[35] In order to "ally ourselves with those who are dedicated to building a society free from oppression," the institute urges therapists to get involved in "public education . . . lobbying for legislative action and other appropriate activities."[36] Some feminist therapists even encourage patients to take political action. "How would you encourage [your patients] to take social and political action?" asks a textbook written for students studying feminist therapy.[37]

Feminist therapy is gaining ground. Graduate training programs in clinical psychology offer specialty tracks in "feminist practice," and university-run student health centers routinely hire feminist therapists to counsel undergraduates. Fledgling clinical psychologists taking the licensing exam are expected to study feminist therapy. The board review preparatory manual of the Association for Advanced Training in the Behavioral Sciences devotes an entire section to it. The American Psychological Association features feminist therapy along with time-honored and well-studied techniques in its information to the public on the kinds of psychotherapies conducted by psychologists.[38]

Multicultural Counseling

Just as feminist therapists think of their patients as battling the patriarchy, multicultural counselors assume that their patients are struggling against racism. Multicultural counseling grew out of civil rights–era efforts to integrate black men into the workforce. A 1950 article published in the *Journal of Clinical Psychology* introduced the topic of psychotherapy for minority patients. Titled "The Negro Patient in Psychotherapy," it raised two perfectly legitimate questions: What is the nature of the relationship between a minority patient and a white therapist he perceives as racist? And can a white therapist respond to a minority patient as an individual rather than as a member of a minority group?[39]

In 1950 the forward-looking goal was to move beyond race and treat all patients as individuals. Today's multicultural counseling, in contrast, argues for treating minority patients as members of a group rather than as unique individuals. Elaine Pinderhughes nicely captures this perspective in her book *Understanding Race, Ethnicity and Power*. A psychiatric social worker, Pinderhughes condemns psychotherapists who practice what she calls a "white, middle-class model of therapy" that "has valued individual responsibility, looking inward, self-understanding and insight, personal growth and change, resolution of dependency needs, verbal and emotional expressiveness and thinking problems through." According to Pinderhughes, "Non-white, non-middle-class cultures" may be more likely to benefit from hands-on approaches, advice-giving and "change efforts directed toward the environment."[40]

Her recommended approach has merits, but those have nothing to do with race. As a psychiatrist working mostly with substance-abusing minority patients in Washington, D.C., I generally emphasize advice-giving aimed at making practical changes in the patient's environment, so as to reduce the stress and boredom that increase the risk of drug use and crime. I did the same thing when I worked in New Haven, Connecticut, where my drug-abusing patients were mostly white.

Like feminist therapy, multicultural counseling promotes activism. At the American Counseling Association (ACA) 1999 world conference in San Diego, many members voiced approval of the move to incorporate social activism into the formal role of the professional counselor. A new division called Counselors for Social Justice recently joined the ACA with the goal of "eradicating oppressive systems of power and privilege [and] the implementation of social action strategies."[41] In 1998 the association published a book called *Social Action: A Mandate for Counselors*.[42]

Activism is not only for therapists but for patients too. In his text-book *Multicultural Therapy,* Manuel Ramirez of the University of Texas at Austin says that the ultimate goal of therapy is to encourage *patients* to become "multicultural ambassadors for the development of a cooperative and peaceful multicultural society."[43] They are to go forth and become "multicultural educators and peer counselors for those who are suffering from feeling different and from mismatch shock." Mismatch shock, according to Ramirez, comes from living in a society that has made one a "victim of conformity or assimilation."[44] I suspect that no matter what a patient tells Ramirez, he will manage to diagnose "mismatch shock."

But before counselors can become activists they must undergo the counseling equivalent of sensitivity training. The "Multicultural Counseling Competencies" devised by the Association for Multicultural Counseling and Development state that "White counselors [must] understand how they may have directly or indirectly benefitted from individual, institutional and cultural racism."[45] The ideal counselors, according to the association, "are constantly seeking to understand themselves as racial and cultural beings and are actively seeking a non-racist identity." Some multicultural practitioners are utterly pessimistic that counselors can help patients unless the counselors themselves first submit to these soul-searching exercises. At the 1998 ACA world conference, Robbie J. Steward and her colleagues at Michigan State University in East Lansing focused on the experiences and attitudes of counselor-trainees. They puzzled aloud over "white trainees who, for reasons we do not quite understand at this time, are perceived as multiculturally competent by minority clients before receiving multicultural counseling training or course work."[46]

Teaching Multicultural Counseling

"My students want to know how to do black therapy, Hispanic therapy and so on," complains Morris L. Jackson of Bowie State University, one of Maryland's historically black colleges. "I certainly don't know what race-based therapy is. What I teach them are principles and basic techniques that apply to human beings—to be respectful, open-minded, curious and caring."[47] Jackson is right. He has taken on an uphill battle trying to persuade the American Counseling Association and his colleagues to soften their race-conscious stance. Multicultural counseling is a rapidly expanding field. In the 1970s and early 1980s, Jackson explained, only a handful of counseling training programs required multicultural counseling courses, but now as many as six in ten programs require such a course, and almost all offer at least one. To obtain licensure at the state level, many states require a course in multicultural counseling. According to the National Board of Counselor Certification, many applicants satisfy the requirement for learning about the "social and cultural foundations of counseling" by taking a multicultural counseling course.[48]

Jackson is dismayed by the attitude of many of his multicultural counselor colleagues who "assume that students who are not minorities are racist, and teach with that assumption in mind." That is the assumption of Allison Cummings-McCann of Emporia State University in Kansas, who urges counselors and trainees to adopt "White awareness" and "unlearn racism."[49] It is also the assumption of David Stone of Northern Illinois University, who frets that counselors are unaware of their social privilege. To be effective counselors, Stone believes, they must "combat the detrimental effects of privilege."[50] The *Journal of Counseling and Development* (the major journal in the field) devoted an entire issue to "privilege" and "oppression" in counseling called "Racism: Healing Its Effects."[51]

Indeed, some counseling programs are literally educating the next generation of therapists to impart their own political worldview to patients. Says Edil Torres Rivera, on the counseling faculty of the University of Nevada at Reno: "Many of my students and clients suffer from living in a sick society."[52] It is hard to imagine how students specializing in multicultural counseling can escape feeling pressure to conform to the political leanings of their teachers. The only way, I fear, is when the trainees walk into grad school on the first day of classes already believing that the dominant culture is the root of psychopathology. By the time they graduate as therapists, these multiculturalists will be so thoroughly schooled in the oppressive ways of society that they'll be able to read bias into virtually anything patients tell them. After all, as an ACA advocacy paper makes clear: "The majority of counselors belong to dominant groups and have been the recipients of less oppression [than their clients]. . . . They are recipients of privilege due to their socio-racial identity in society and within the profession; they have influence due to their numerical majority."[53]

The textbooks, too, assume that racism infects trainees. *Counseling the Culturally Different* asks the reader, "As a member of the White group, what responsibility do you hold for the racist, oppressive, and discriminating manner by which you personally and professionally deal with minorities?" The textbook's authors insist that "without a strong anti-racism training component, trainees (especially Whites) will continue to deny responsibility for the racist system that oppresses their minority clients."[54]

This encourages impressionable trainees to expect that minority patients will be hostile. It also inculcates the kind of guilt-ridden attitude manifested by "Paul," a subscriber to the multicultural counseling list serve: "While it remains important to bring experiences of oppressed people to the fore, I believe this must be balanced by engaging members of privileged groups in a conversation about their roles and responsibilities regarding [homophobia and heterosexism]. . . . I, as a white person . . . must identify racism as my disease as I am part of an institution that gains power by it."[55]

This is just the kind of sentiment that prompted Robert E. Wubbolding, professor of counseling at Xavier University in Ohio, to remark, "I am convinced that the multicultural movement is largely negative. I suggest graduate students ask their professors to spend at least as much time on the positive aspects of society as they do on racism, bigotry and prejudice."[56] How can counselors help their patients overcome outlooks that are bleak and hopeless, Wubbolding wonders, if young counselors are being trained to see patients as set upon by such dark societal forces? "I can't think of a better way to hold minorities back than to teach that everyone is biased, prejudiced, racist and bigoted. It engenders an 'I can't' worldview in clients," he says.

Another problem with multicultural counseling is that it often requires the acceptance of blatant ethnic stereotypes. Consider the following examples from textbooks on multicultural counseling:

- The worldview of the culturally different client boils down to one important question: "What makes you any different from all the others out there who have oppressed and discriminated against me?"[57]

- The Asian American's "greater social awareness causes him/her to be somewhat more sensitive to racism and to often react with overt anger or militance."[58]

- "Time is not a fundamental variable [for Hispanics]; do not ask a [Hispanic] client reasons for being late to therapy."[59]

- "Avoid linking mental problems [of African Americans] to parents' behaviors; these problems result from environmental conflicts in society."[60]

Culture, of course, has a considerable influence on personal identity, but it is only one influence among a great many, and it does not predictably determine the nature of one's distress nor the formula for its amelioration. By evaluating cultural influences the same way they evaluate every other influence—individually, one patient at a time—therapists can avoid the confusion that is the inevitable by-product of the group stereotyping found in various textbooks. To some degree, of course, all counseling relationships are "cross-cultural" relationships. No person can fully "know" the reality of another's life, no matter how similar their lives may be in outward appearance.

A student named Regina innocently succumbed to that confusion. Here is the message she posted on the diversity counseling list serve that I was on.

> I am a graduate student in a counseling program. . . . Is it difficult to work with [a patient] whose values and beliefs may be unknown or completely different from yours? I have a dilemma. I have lived long enough in the Middle East, Italy, Belgium, Poland, and other countries so that I consider myself an individual with a multicultural background. Every client in my caseload will be an individual with a different background from my own. Do you

think it will be possible for me to be an effective counselor with such a background?[61]

Regina's query epitomizes what multiculturalism in therapy has wrought. Here we have a dedicated student with a wonderful breadth of cultural and linguistic experiences who has been made to worry needlessly. *There must be some counseling formula I can memorize,* she is thinking, *that will tell me what to do if my ethnic background is A and my client's ethnic background is B.* If so, Regina is doomed. After all, every client belongs to numerous groups. "It does not take much imagination to recognize that the number of combinations and permutations of these groups is staggering," notes C. H. Patterson, emeritus professor of counseling at the University of Illinois.[62]

Indeed, as Patterson points out, attempting to develop different theories, methods and techniques for each of these groups would be an insurmountable task. Why haven't Regina's professors taught her that the individual, with his unique emotions, cognitions, actions and spirituality, is the focus of counseling, not the group to which he belongs? Why hasn't she learned that a keen interest in her patients and her kindness to them transcend the specifics of culture? How helpful is the multicultural perspective, we may ask, if it obscures the true purpose of therapy: to help patients observe themselves, understand and take responsibility for their choices and appreciate how they unwittingly get in the way of their own happiness and accomplishment.

The 2000 American Counseling Association Convention

"The ACA allows multicultural therapy to be a front for a political agenda," Stephen Weinrach, professor of counseling at Villanova University, told an audience at the 2000 ACA annual meeting in Washington, D.C.[63] Therapy should be devoted to self-determination, Weinrach emphasized, not to cataloging the ways in which the client has been held back, not to urging him to pursue social redress. Self-awareness is not a by-product of activism; if anything, activism takes the focus off the patient. Victim politics, he said, has "hijacked the profession of counseling; propaganda about social justice now dominates our journals, our textbooks, our curriculum and our conventions."

The 2000 convention, which I attended, offered dozens of seminars on social justice and race-consciousness. In one, called "Promoting Social Justice Through Counselor Education," the audience was instructed to attend to the "advocacy needs of the community."[64] One example given was marching against welfare reform. Another seminar focused on "the growing awareness of how various forms of social injustice and oppression impact clients' mental health." Counselors were exhorted to address the racism and sexism that "continue to be perpetuated in our society."[65]

Such practical matters, however, are not what many multicultural counselors have in mind. According to list-serve member Chris, counselors should get involved, in their role as counselors (rather than as concerned citizens), with issues such as "misuse of nuclear power," "consumer exploitation," "ecological abuse" and the "technological obsolescence of American workers."[66]

Admittedly, a therapist must sometimes assume a directive role. Many times the clinician needs to make the first move to jump-start a reluctant patient on the path to taking charge. When one of my patients said that she was molested by a male nurse in a local emergency room but was uneasy about reporting him, I put her in touch with the hospital ombudsman. She then went on to pursue her charge of abuse. Another patient couldn't read and was too embarrassed to do something about it. I helped her contact an agency that would teach her to read.

One must be careful, of course, not to let the patient feel too comfortable and to assume that the therapist will step in and take care of things. A posture of rescuing the patient has risks, as Professor Clemmont Vontress of the American University notes: "The problems presented by many clients cause some counselors to feel that they somehow must do for them what [the clients'] parents [and] teachers have been unable to do."[67]

Not only are counselors, textbooks and the profession itself biased in the eyes of multicultural counselors, but the patients themselves must be assessed for signs of bigotry as well. According to Julie Ancis of Georgia State University in Atlanta, counselors must attend to their "clients' prejudicial attitudes and discriminatory behaviors."[68] If they don't, Ancis warned an audience at the 2000 ACA conference, their patients' psychological difficulties will never be resolved; they are, after all, linked to their bigoted attitudes and behaviors, she said. I wondered how patients' personal prejudices were linked to the reasons they sought counseling—to improve a marriage, to become more assertive, to come to terms with a loss.

The association required convention speakers to discuss diversity issues. If you wanted to organize one of the special full- or half-day training sessions during the three-day event, you had to first submit a written statement to the ACA attesting to the following:

- Your knowledge level of culture/diversity–related information on the topic you were proposing

- Steps you would take to avoid presenting stereotypical imagery

- The nature and relevance of the case examples you would use, including universal, or lack of universal, applications of the cases across cultures[69]

It was the naive speaker, alas, who resisted this assault on his professional autonomy. The association asked everyone in the audience to fill out an evaluation form and to rate the speaker on such things as "openness to discussing and answering questions on diversity/culture issues."[70]

Patients as Casualties

Multicultural counseling has not been put to any kind of test. Few, if any, of the multicultural counseling "experts" have demonstrated their techniques at professional meetings or videotaped them (as is the collegial tradition in clinical practice), let alone empirically validated them.[71] I could find no controlled studies of patients wherein half are randomly assigned to multicultural counseling and half to conventional counseling. Such research, of course, would first require that multicultural counseling be defined and operationalized, a task its proponents have yet to undertake.

Nonetheless, it is clear that one of the defining elements of multicultural counseling is the instillation of race-consciousness. A number of my colleagues have told me of clinic directors who insist that black patients can be treated only by black counselors.

Others concede that perhaps the counselors need not be black, but that the patients must still be educated in oppression. For example, the federal Center for Substance Abuse Prevention produced a booklet called *An African-Centered Model of Prevention for African-American Youth at High Risk.*[72] The essays in the booklet say that black youngsters must first be made aware of their oppression if they are to avoid or overcome addiction, gang involvement and teen pregnancy. A West Dallas program for nine- to twelve-year-olds is described in the booklet. As part of substance abuse prevention education, the students are taught Afrocentric myth: "Youths are taken through a study of African history. . . . They [learn about] Africa as the origin of architecture . . . astronomy . . . mathematics and libraries."[73]

When Lauretta Omeltschenko worked as a counselor in residential programs for addicted women in the Midwest, Afrocentrism was a big part of the treatment programs. "One program focused its curriculum heavily on racial issues," Omeltschenko says. "The African American staff encouraged African dress, African values and Kwanzaa." Another program put the black patients on a van once a week and sent them off to "black pride, empowerment and recovery meeting, whether or not they wanted to go," she tells me. Typically, about half the black patients objected to the African themes. Omeltschenko says, "They would say, 'Kwanzaa isn't African, it was made up in the sixties by an American,' or, 'My skin color has nothing to do with my recovery.'"[74]

Meant to elevate their self-esteem by emphasizing black pride, the sessions ended up instructing the women in how they had been victims of racism, which many found a silly distraction, Omeltschenko says. But unfortunately, some used the lessons about oppression as a wedge issue. "The supposed fascism of the white staff and some of the other white patients became something else for the black patients to focus on," she notes. "The women should have been working on their addiction and other problems, but instead we spent many hours on pointless, divisive arguing about who discriminated against whom." Worse, a number of the counselors encouraged the patients to view the social dynamics of the residential program through the lens of race.

Omeltschenko's description of group process reminds me of my tenure as a staff psychiatrist on inpatient wards. Like her residential program, these wards often emphasized cooperation within a community of patients as an essential part of the therapy. We knew that the frequent efforts of patients to blame staff and other patients were usually a way to divert attention from the hard work of changing themselves. We were constantly pointing this out to them; that was part of the therapy. This technique works only when the entire staff shares basic assumptions about therapy; otherwise, the patients can play them off against each other. Omeltschenko herself eventually became so frustrated trying to protect patients from being inculated about their victimhood—and being forced to hire underqualified staff to meet racial quotas—that she quit.

I too encountered Afrocentric themes in counseling during my tenure as a staff psychiatrist for the superior court in Washington, D.C. Our patients had committed minor crimes to maintain a drug habit and had been court-ordered to drug treatment. Almost all were African American, most of them in their twenties and thirties. On a daily basis most of their clinical contact was with counselors who believed that self-esteem was the key to success. Somehow the patients were supposed to absorb self-esteem by participating in Afrocentric exercises, not from achieving anything in particular. There were "group therapies" in which the men used crayons to color in stencils of the African continent. Meanwhile, a good fraction of the men were illiterate or did not have a GED. Most of the other patients, even if they had a GED or high school diploma, had no technical skills.

And that was what they wanted. To a man, each wanted to get a GED or learn a trade like plumbing or electrical wiring and join a union. They were struggling to be polite when I asked them what they thought of the program: "Mickey Mouse" and "a waste of our time" were common characterizations. The clinic director and I wanted to bring in tutors and even set up apprenticeships in plumbing and carpentry for some patients. The counselors, for their part, did not lift a finger to help. If the situation wasn't depressing enough, our patients had no choice but to remain in a third-rate program. They were court-ordered to that particular one. To be sure, the fact that they were required to attend was a blessing. That precious opportunity was squandered, however, on feel-good exercises conducted by multiculturally oriented counselors.

Ironically, the ACA "Code of Ethics" appears to proscribe much of what multicultural counselors are doing. The code specifically says that "counselors should avoid imposing their values on clients" and that they "should avoid exploiting the trust and dependency of clients."[75] To treat patients with the intention of getting them involved in social activism and teaching them to assume roles as multicultural "educators" and "ambassadors" is a gross violation of these codes. "The job is not a bully pulpit to further our own social agenda," says Professor Brian S. Canfield of the University of Louisiana at Monroe.[76] "Counselors should always respond to the issues presented by the client," says Clemmont Vontress of American University, "not the issues which trouble them, the counselors."[77]

Nowadays multicultural counselors who work on college campuses must feel right at home. After all, campuses are ground-zero for the excesses of political correctness. Many assume that the era of speech codes is over, collapsed of its own ludicrous and Orwellian weight. But they are wrong. In *The Shadow University,* Alan Kors and Harvey Silverglate describe racism eradication exercises that are required for entering freshmen. A central goal of these programs is to root out "internalized oppression," as elaborated in the education planning documents of most universities.

> At Wake Forest University [in 1999], one of the few events designated as "mandatory" for freshman orientation was attendance at Blue Eyed, a filmed racism awareness workshop in which whites are abused, ridiculed, made to fail, and taught helpless passivity so

that they can identify with "a person of color for a day." In Swarthmore College's dormitories, in the fall of 1998, first-year students were asked to line up by skin color, from lightest to darkest, and to step forward and talk about how they felt concerning their place in that line. Indeed, at almost all of our campuses, some form of moral and political re-education has been built into freshman orientation and residential programming.

These exercises have become so "commonplace that most students do not even think of the issues of privacy, rights, and dignity involved," say Alan Charles Kors, professor of history at the University of Pennsylvania.[78] Is it too far-fetched to wonder whether an insufficiently apologetic freshman would be sent to a multicultural therapist for a more intensive, private session of racism eradication?

Sexual Disorientation

Homosexuals also have a place on the multicultural therapist's couch. Kelley, a graduate student in counseling, thinks that her colleagues must appreciate the existence of a homosexual culture. "In order to effectively counsel gay men and lesbians, one needs to recognize that their experiences living in our society may be different from other clients' experiences," she writes on my diversity list serve.[79] Will Kelley reflexively fixate on "heterosexism" as the cause of unhappiness in her gay patients? She might decide to get special credentialing from the Chicago Center for Family Health, home of the country's first certificate program for LBGT (lesbian, bisexual, gay and transsexual) counseling.[80]

Kelley is right that homosexuals have "experiences" different from those of straight people by virtue of their same-sex attraction. But the personal meaning of these experiences is unique, shaped by the myriad strivings, conflicts, fears and wishes that each homosexual person, indeed all of us, harbors. Recognizing this should not require special training on the part of the therapist. In fact, formal certification risks ghettoizing the mental health needs of gay people and creates the illusion that special knowledge is required. This could lead a patient to deny himself care by a perfectly competent but "uncertified" therapist. Conversely, it could lead young therapists to think that perhaps they are unqualified and hence to turn away patients whom they could truly help.

A good therapist elicits each patient's one-of-a-kind constellation of thoughts and emotions—a veritable psychic fingerprint—and in doing so creates conditions for the patient to show how he sees himself and the world and to tell what he thinks he needs. One of those needs may be to clarify his sexual orientation. Though the nature-nurture debate surrounding homosexuality is unresolved, it is fair to say that same-sex attraction and gay or lesbian identity exist along a continuum. At one pole are individuals with a strong biological predisposition; at the other are individuals who have deliberately chosen a gay or lesbian lifestyle. Many other men and women fall somewhere in between. Inhabitants of that middle ground who are living as gay may be ambivalent about their sexual orientation. Some seek psychological help to resolve that ambivalence—some with the goal of feeling more comfortable as homosexual, others with the intention of exploring heterosexuality.

Both goals are clinically valid, and some—though by no means all— of the patients who have set out to achieve them have been successful. Nonetheless, the treatment of ambivalent men and women who seek to "convert" to heterosexuality has sparked angry debate among therapists. "All mental health professional organizations take issue with those who claim success in 'healing' gay men and lesbians," proclaims Bob Barret, former president of the Association for Gay, Lesbian and Bisexual Issues in Counseling.[81] Other counselors have called such therapy "prejudicial," suggesting that therapists want to convert unsuspecting patients because of their own homophobia.[82]

The accusations of prejudice, however, go both ways. The American Psychological Association, for example, says on its general information web site that sexual orientation is never a choice and that therapy cannot change it.[83] Richard Isay of the American Psychiatric Association's Committee on Gay, Lesbian and Bisexual Issues calls therapists who have treated gay men and lesbians who wish to assume a heterosexual lifestyle "abusers of psychiatry."[84] The National Association of Social Workers issued an official statement denouncing so-called conversion therapy (also called reparative therapy) and discouraging social workers from referring patients to therapists who are willing to see patients for that purpose.[85]

For men and women confused about their sexuality, the battle over conversion therapy only heightens their anxiety. If they are unlucky enough to encounter a prejudiced therapist of either variety—one who thinks homosexuality is a pathology to be cured or one who is too closed-minded to acknowledge the mutability of sexuality—their genuine desire to explore themselves and even change (or maintain) their sexual behaviors will be stifled in the name of gender politics.

San Francisco General Hospital

San Francisco General Hospital, the major teaching hospital of the University of California at San Francisco, is home to the most prominent multicultural program in the country. Now called the Cultural Competence and Diversity Program, it began in the 1970s when the hospital created a specialty ward for Asian patients to address the language barrier faced by many recent immigrants seeking mental health services. By centralizing staff members who spoke Asian languages, the hospital found that it could improve service—indeed, what little quality research has been done on some forms of multicultural therapy has found that overcoming language barriers is probably the only significant benefit. A few years later a similar program was started for non-English-speaking Hispanic patients; it too was a successful effort to extend care to underserved populations.[86]

But victim politics soon replaced the language barrier as the rationale for specially designed treatment. African Americans, gays and women also wanted their own units (or "teams," as they were called). Today each new patient admitted to the psychiatric service at San Francisco General is assigned to a treatment team specializing in one of six specific groups—African Americans, Asians, Latinos, gays/lesbians/bisexuals, women and HIV-positive individuals. Each team is guided by a "curriculum," which specifies the proper procedures for treating members of the group. Although staff members and patients are not rigidly segregated by group, I was told by the head of the psychiatry service that the hospital does make an effort to have at least half the staff and patients on any given team be homogeneous.[87] The only patients without a team dedicated to them are white male heterosexuals.

The Black Focus Team is a striking example of multicultural therapy. Merely in order to qualify for a job on the team, some nurses, social workers, orderlies and other nonphysician staff members have to be certified by the San Francisco Civil Service Commission as "African American Health Specialists." The certification process, from which black employees were *not* exempted, entails taking a thirty-two-hour course on African American health services and logging "1,000 work hours of direct health-related service hours to African-American clients."[88] This requirement implies that, absent special training, certain health professionals are unqualified to care for African American patients.

Much of the effort on the Black Focus Team is directed toward reeducating the nonblack staff, who are assumed to harbor racist attitudes. As the curriculum explains, "All of us have been raised in a racist world, inundated by myths, distortions, and stereotypes of black people." Accordingly, one of the "educational objectives" for the team's staff is to "break down denial of one's own participation in racism." Michelle Clark, psychiatrist and head of the Black Focus Team, explains that "we work with our staff not to be afraid to engage in the kinds of dyads that historically might have led to legal action or possibly even damage or death, such as to have a white woman [a nurse] speaking to a black man [a patient]."[89]

This hypersensitivity to race is not without risk. A few years ago it led to problems between the mostly black staff and the psychiatric residents, most of whom are white or Asian. Relations grew so unbearably tense that several years ago Robert Okin, the chief of psychiatry, stopped assigning first-year residents to the team. Several of the residents described to me an "anti-white atmosphere," and one former Asian resident reported feeling "blamed, somehow, for the patients' problems." Another pointed out that, ironically, most of the patients were so psychotic that they were oblivious to the identity politics.

Racism as a Mental Illness?

Alvin F. Poussaint, a Harvard psychiatrist, takes the relationship between racism and pathology one step further. He argues that the racist individual is mentally ill. In a *New York Times* op-ed piece ("They Hate. They Kill. Are They Insane?"), Poussaint asserted that extreme racism should be classified as a mental illness and listed alongside disorders such as major depression and schizophrenia in the *Diagnostic and Statistical Manual of Mental Disorders*.[90] His commentary was prompted when the white supremacist Buford O. Furrow Jr. opened fire in Los Angeles on children in a Jewish community center and murdered an Asian American man in August 1999.

The plea to designate racial bigotry a mental disease was first made to the American Psychiatric Association by a group of black psychiatrists, including Poussaint, in the wake of racially motivated killings during the civil rights era. The association officials were not receptive—but only because, Poussaint says, "it hasn't been a mental health issue for *them*."[91] To pathologize racism, he told a reporter, would require the association's majority white membership "to look at their friends, their relatives and themselves" in an uncomfortable light. Perhaps such scrutiny would indeed be uncomfortable for some people—for highlighting a moral lapse, however, not a mental deficiency. If anything, turning racism into an illness would soften the stigma of being a bigot and open the door for all kinds of exculpatory legal defenses—hardly the consequences that Poussaint has in mind.

Yet he maintains that anyone who wants to eliminate blacks, or Jews, or whites, in the belief that they are responsible for the world's troubles, "meets criteria for delusional disorder, a major psychiatric illness." Not true. Psychiatry defines a delusion as an irrational idea that is not ordinarily accepted by other members of the patient's culture or subculture. Furrow's neo-Nazi vision, offensive as it might be, is shared by other people. It is not evidence of psychosis. Nor is racism the only example of shared irrationality in our culture. Others include "an uncritical belief in telepathy, alien abduction, and reincarnation, to name a few," says Robert

L. Spitzer, a professor of psychiatry at Columbia University. "The last thing that psychiatry or society in general needs is to confuse the distinction between the sometimes overlapping concepts of evil, crackpot and mental illness."[92]

Colin Ferguson, the schizophrenic black man who gunned down white commuters on the Long Island Railroad in 1994, was the embodiment of insanity. He killed because he was psychotic about whites. He also harbored other delusions and symptoms that typically respond to antipsychotic medication. Other mass killers who hate, like Timothy McVeigh, are not psychotic. Their ideas are part of their character, not an illness. No medication can change their desire to destroy other people.

The Atlanta Braves pitcher John Rocker revealed some of his character in the December 1999 issue of *Sports Illustrated*. There he made disparaging remarks about immigrants, homosexuals and a black teammate. Before disciplining Rocker, Major League Baseball Commissioner Bud Selig first wanted to hear from mental health professionals. He required Rocker to undergo psychiatric evaluation, a neo-Orwellian maneuver implying that anyone who uses bigoted language may well be mentally ill. "John Rocker is a jerk," wrote the columnist and psychiatrist Charles Krauthammer, "but jerk is not a medical diagnosis."[93] Indeed, the commissioner—like Poussaint—sought to medicalize ideas and actions that we rightly object to on moral grounds.

Poussaint's bid to make violent racism a mental illness, the baseball commissioner's implication that bigotry is evidence of psychopathology and the efforts of multicultural counselors to treat the "victims" of discrimination show how racism has become an all-purpose pathogen. Like a virus, it sickens the carrier, whose actions go on to cause pathology in others. This is a powerful social metaphor for the corrosive effects of hatred, but it is meaningless in the realm of health.

The Oppression Obsessions

The common assumption linking the three forms of therapy explored in this chapter is that patients' problems must first be understood as the result of outside forces if their psychological health is to be restored. A helpless child, to be sure, can fairly blame his abuser for harm done, but a therapist's preoccupation with the traumatic experiences of childhood is unlikely to help a fragile adult patient get better. As we saw in Maine, it can even cause patients to regress.

Naturally, some people can be helped by understanding the relationship between their current problems and a traumatic past. The patient who rewrites the script of his life so that it has more meaning, or angles the prism of memory until he is at peace, can achieve a profound sense of well-being. But it is not a task for impulsive people who slit their wrists, who can't hold a job, who have few friends, who are erratic or who use drugs. They have more pressing matters to attend to, like relating to their families, learning how to hold a job and finding strategies for making it responsibly through the day.

What's more, deep psychotherapy can bring up feelings and stir recollections that overwhelm people who are not adept at handling anxiety. That's why, for example, I strongly discourage psychotherapy for a recovering addict who has not been clean and sober for at least a year.

Nor does encouraging patients to think of themselves as victims of sexism or racism help them overcome their problems. It is the therapist's job to help the patient explore a range of possible explanations for her difficulties. This is not to deny that discrimination exists and that patients may be affected by it. If the patient has indeed suffered from bias, the therapist should help her consider a range of constructive responses to it—that is, responses that don't sabotage the patient's own well-being. If the patient decides she wants redress, then she should be advised by an ombudsman, a lawyer or an advocacy group.

In general, oppression-based therapies are enormously seductive because they tend to absolve the sufferer of responsibility. This is precisely why therapists should not practice them. After all, the virtue of therapy is that it takes a person from thinking of himself as a victim to one who is an agent of his own destiny. Emphasizing social injustice as the sole source of distress reinforces self-pity and anger, depriving patients of the opportunity to improve their lives through self-knowledge.

The anecdotal cases I have uncovered are probably the tip of the iceberg. While I am certain that the competent therapists outnumber the radicals, there are so many indoctrinologists seated at the helm of the ACA and, to a lesser extent, the American Psychological Association that a serious challenge to these trends will probably not be mounted anytime soon. Given the politicized agenda of feminist therapy and multicultural counseling, the imposition of the therapists' worldview on patients and the assault on introspection, I think one can make the case that the most radical forms of these therapies constitute nothing less than malpractice.

Epilogue

The Indoctrinologist Isn't In . . . Yet

INDOCTRINOLOGISTS ARE MAKING STEADY INROADS in medicine. They now sit at the helm of professional associations and hold impressive posts in schools of public health. They have changed medical school admissions criteria and have infiltrated respected academic journals. They are outspoken, if not shrill, participants in many legislative and political debates. Although practitioners of PC medicine do not constitute a majority in the health professions, their numbers and influence are growing. Most disturbing, their stubborn reluctance to acknowledge each person's responsibility in preserving his own health threatens to reverse many of the gains made by the public health movement in the past century.

The general public is largely unaware of the existence of indoctrinologists. And because their activities are spread over many areas of medicine—from nursing to psychotherapy to schools of public health—it isn't easy to measure their reach or describe their efforts tidily. Nonetheless, those who care about the culture and practice of medicine must be alert to the encroachment of political agendas that are diverting resources from vital clinical tasks.

Some of the more absurd manifestations of PC medicine can be reversed overnight. Federal and state governments should cease funding consumer-survivor groups, for example, and nursing school deans should cancel therapeutic touch courses. Feminist and multicultural "practitioners" should not be hired by agencies and clinics that provide mental health services.

These steps would be a good first move, but they are unlikely to disarm the politically correct troops whose mission is nothing less than the reinvention of modern medical practice. Even harder to reform will be the universities, where many forms of political correctness, such as racial preferences in admission, have been thriving for some time. While the medical schools' goal of recruiting more minority doctors is admirable, group-based preferences that debase standards of excellence are bad medicine for patients and physicians alike. Similarly, our schools of public health, once wellsprings of practical innovation and discovery, now advance an ideologically driven agenda that claims disease to be the product of oppression.

It is easy for purveyors of PC medicine to see malign social forces (sexism, classism, racism) and corrupt institutions (patriarchal medicine, biased doctors, authoritarian psychiatry) in any measurable health disparity. After all, they are steeped in a Marcusian worldview in which the power elite will do anything to maintain their control, even if this means compromising the physical or mental status of vulnerable people or betraying the truth about health risks.

We must remain clear-eyed about the fact that uneven access to medical services, disparate knowledge of good health practices and personal attitudes—not discrimination and bias—underlie the vast majority of differences in health outcomes. Moreover, health professionals must concentrate on the problems that they can actually do something about: preventing and alleviating the nation's physical—not its social—distress. And though it may be fashionable to blame our ills on oppression or alienation, the reality is far more complicated. It is true that health is not solely in the hands of individuals. There is an undeniable need for systemic improvements to the nation's health care system. But each of us can and must play a role in maintaining our own health.

Fortunately, there are built-in limits to the corrupting influence of PC medicine. Our society has come to expect and continues to demand technical excellence in health care, and thus far the medical profession has provided it. Most men and women in medical practice are people of integrity, too dedicated to caring for the sick to be swayed by a politicized agenda. Most scientists will not compromise rigor for the sake of promoting victim politics. Most public health professionals want to extend the proud work of their discipline, not make political statements.

Curbing the destructive tendencies of PC medicine demands that health care practitioners and researchers embolden themselves to defend standards of excellence and professionalism. The public also needs to be alerted to the crisis. Together, clinicians, researchers and the public can inoculate medicine against the life-or-death consequences of political correctness.

Notes

Introduction

1. Sue Poole, "Where Should Dollars Go?: Voluntary Community Support," MadNation, http://www.madnation.org/tools/needs.htm.

2. Quoted in Robin Marantz Henig, *The People's Health: A Memoir of Public Health and Its Evolution at Harvard* (Washington, DC: Joseph Henry Press, 1997), 15.

3. Sally Zierler, remarks at the annual meeting of the American Public Health Association, Washington, DC, November 16, 1998.

4. Sally Zierler and Nancy Krieger, "Reframing Women's Risk: Social Inequalities and HIV Infection," *Annual Review of Public Health* 18 (1997): 401–36, 417.

Chapter 1

1. Nigel Paneth, Peter Vinten-Johansen, Howard Brody, and Michael Rip, "A Rivalry of Foulness: Official and Unofficial Investigations of the London Cholera Epidemic of 1854," *American Journal of Public Health* 88 (1998): 1545–53.

2. As quoted in T. Pincus, R. Esther, D. A. DeWalt, and L. F. Callahan, "Social Conditions and Self-Management Are More Powerful Determinants of Health Than Access to Care," *Annals of Internal Medicine* 129 (1998): 406–11.

3. Paul Gross and Norman Levitt, *Higher Superstition: The Academic Left and Its Quarrels with Science* (Baltimore: Johns Hopkins University Press, 1994).

4. Robert G. Evans, Morris L. Barer, and Theodore R. Marmor, eds., *Why Are Some People Healthy and Others Not?* (New York: Aldine DeGruyter Press, 1994), 6.

5. Sally Zierler, speaking on the panel "Inequality in Context: Studying the Effect of Neighborhood Conditions and Social Policies on Socioeconomic and Racial/Ethnic Disparities in Health" at the 126th annual meeting of the American Public Health Association, Washington, DC, November 16, 1998.

6. Paul Starr, *The Social Transformation of American Medicine* (New York: Basic Books, 1982), 192.

7. Heather Mac Donald, "Public Health Quackery," *City Journal* (Autumn 1998): 47.

8. Thomas Sowell, *The Quest for Cosmic Justice* (New York: Free Press, 1999), 80.

9. Paula Braverman, "Methods in Health Services Research—Measuring Social Class in Public Health Research: Theoretical, Empirical and Practical Issues," remarks during session 1053.1 at the 124th annual meeting of the American Public Health Association, New York, November 18, 1996.

10. Richard G. Wilkinson, "Income Distribution and Life Expectancy," *British Medical Journal* 304 (1992): 165–68. The theory is also called "social determinants of disease"; see S. Leonard Syme and Jennifer L. Balfour, "Social Determinants of Disease," in *Public Health and Preventive Medicine*, edited by Robert B. Wallace (New York: McGraw-Hill, 1998), 795–810.

11. Ichiro Kawachi, Bruce P. Kennedy, and Richard G. Wilkinson, eds., *The Society and Population Health Reader: Income Inequality and Health* (New York: New Press, 1999), xxxv.

12. Rodney Clark, Norman B. Anderson, Vernessa R. Clark, and David R. Williams, "Racism as a Stressor for African Americans: A Biopsychosocial Model," *American Psychologist* 54, no. 10 (1999): 805–16.

13. Richard S. Cooper, "Health and the Social Status of Blacks in the United States," *Annals of Epidemiology* 3, no. 2 (1993): 137–44.

14. Hortensia Amaro, "HIV Can Be Stopped!" World AIDS Day symposium, sponsored by the Harvard AIDS Institute, Boston, December 1995, http://www.tstradio.com/harpg2.html.

15. Sally Zierler and Nancy Krieger, "Reframing Women's Risk: Social Inequalities and HIV Infection," *Annual Review of Public Health* 18 (1997): 401–36, 417.

16. Nancy Krieger, letter to the editor, *Wall Street Journal,* January 13, 1997; the text of Krieger's letter was posted on the *Wall Street Journal* bulletin board, http://persephone.hampshire.edu/~lists/-minhlth/ msg00669.html, December 15, 1996.

17. Gladys H. Reynolds, "Foreword to the American College of Epidemiology Tenth Annual Scientific Meeting Proceedings," *Annals of Epidemiology* 3, no. 2 (1993): 119.

18. R. A. Hahn, S. M. Teutsch, R. B. Rothenberg, and J. S. Marks, "Excess Deaths from Nine Chronic Diseases in the United States, 1986," *Journal of the American Medical Association* 264 (1990): 2654–59. Hahn and his colleagues (who are from the CDC) report that 52 percent of all deaths in the United States in 1986 were attributable to stroke, coronary heart disease, diabetes, chronic obstructive pulmonary disease, lung cancer, breast cancer, colorectal cancer and chronic liver disease. Many of these deaths, they write, were preventable. The modifiable risk factors include smoking, alcohol abuse, sedentary lifestyle, obesity, high cholesterol and failure to use screening techniques such as mammography and Pap smears. When I spoke to Dr. Hahn on May 22, 2000, he confirmed that this conclusion about preventable deaths remains valid fourteen years later. Also note that the CDC estimates that more than 80 percent of the excess mortality observed among minorities ("excess" means the amount that exceeds that observed among whites) is due to seven causes: cancer, cardiovascular disease and stroke, substance abuse, diabetes, accidents, homicide, infant mortality and AIDS. The course of most, though not all, of these conditions is modifiable by the individual, and substance abuse is a completely self-directed activity; see www.cdc.gov-/od/admn/health.htm.

19. Quoted in Associated Press, "Risk of Death in Men with High Blood Pressure Is Found to Vary by Region," *New York Times,* January 6, 2000; Meir J. Stampfer, Frank B. Hu, JoAnn E. Manson, et al., "Primary Prevention of Coronary Heart Disease in Women Through Diet and Lifestyle," *New England Journal of Medicine* 343 (2000): 16–22.

20. Mindy Thompson-Fullilove, "Abandoning 'Race' as a Variable in Public Health Research—An Idea Whose Time Has Come," *American Journal of Public Health* 88, no. 9 (1998): 1297–98, 1298.

21. Vincent Iacopino, remarks during the 124th annual meeting of the American Public Health Association, New York, November 17–21, 1996.

22. Deborah Prothrow-Stith, M.D., undated statement distributed at the annual meeting of the American Public Health Association, New York, November 17–21, 1996.

23. Philip Cole, Elizabeth Delzell, and Brad Rodu, "Moneychangers in the Temple," *Epidemiology* 11, no. 1 (2000): 84–90.

24. Mary Anne Mercer, letter to APHA Governing Council members, October 26, 1996.

25. Sally Zierler, speaking on the panel "Inequality in Context: Studying Effects of Neighborhood Conditions and Social Policies on Socioeconomic and Racial/Ethnic Disparities in Health" at the 126th annual meeting of the American Public Health Association, Washington, DC, November 16, 1998.

26. David G. Whiteis, *Chronicle of Higher Education* online colloquy, http://chronicle.com/colloquy/99/ormh/.03.htm, response posted September 7, 1999.

27. Robert Beaglehole and Ruth Bonita, *Public Health at the Crossroads: Achievements and Prospects* (New York: Cambridge University Press, 1997).

28. C.-E. A. Winslow, "The Untilled Fields of Public Health," *Science* 51 (1920): 20–31, 30.

29. Institute of Medicine, *The Future of Public Health* (Washington, DC: National Academy Press, 1988), 40. "Unfortunately," write the sympathetic authors of *Public Health at the Crossroads*, "for many epidemiologists the study of social factors is considered too political"; see Robert Beaglehole and Ruth Bonita, *Public Health at the Crossroads: Achievements and Prospects* (New York: Cambridge University Press, 1997), 120.

30. Carl M. Shy, "The Failure of Academic Epidemiology: Witness for the Prosecution," *American Journal of Epidemiology* 145 (1997): 479–84.

31. Quoted in Robin Marantz Henig, *The People's Health: A Memoir of Public Health and Its Evolution at Harvard* (Washington, DC: Joseph Henry Press, 1997), 4.

32. Lawrence Wallack and Lori Dorfman, "Media Advocacy: A Strategy for Advancing Policy and Promoting Health," *Health Education Quarterly* 23, no. 3 (1996): 293–317.

33. Quoted in ibid., 15.

34. Barbara A. Israel, Amy J. Schulz, Edith A. Parker, and Adam B. Becker, "Review of Community-Based Research: Assessing Partnership Approaches to Improve Public Health," *Annual Review of Public Health* 19 (1998): 172–202, 179.

35. Ernest T. Stringer, *Action Research: Handbook for Practitioners* (Thousand Oaks, CA: Sage Publications, 1996), x.

36. M. Douglas Anglin, personal communication with the author, May 9, 1999.

37. Meredith Minkler and Nina Wallerstein, "Improving Health Through Community Organizing and Community Building: A Health Education Perspective," in *Community Organizing and Community Building for Health,* edited by Meredith Minkler (New Brunswick, NJ: Rutgers University Press, 1998), 30–52, 40.

38. Cole, Delzell, and Rodu, "Moneychangers in the Temple," 87.

39. Donald E. Waite, D.O., letter to the author, January 10, 2000.

40. This is the accusation (accurate in my view) made by the counsel for the defense in Carl Shy's mock courtroom in Shy, "The Failure of Academic Epidemiology: Witness for the Prosecution."

41. Kenneth Rothman, Hans-Olov Adami, and Dimitrios Trichopoulos, "Should the Mission of Epidemiology Include the Eradication of Poverty?" *Lancet* 352 (1998): 810–13, 812.

42. Trude Bennett and Raj Bhopal, "Survey of Editorial Policy on Race and Ethnicity Research," abstract distributed at the American Public Health Association meeting, Indianapolis, IN, November 9–13, 1997.

43. Committee on Minority Affairs, "Statement of Principles, Epidemiology and Minority Populations" (approved by full board of the American College of Epidemiology), *Annals of Epidemiology* 5 (1995): 505–8.

44. David A. Savitz, personal communication with the author, August 5, 1999.

45. Alexander M. Walker, "'Kangaroo Court': Invited Commentary on Shy's 'The Failure of Academic Epidemiology: Witness for the Prosecution,'" *American Journal of Epidemiology* 145 (1997): 485–86.

46. Deborah Cohen, Suzanne Spear, Richard Scribner, et al., "'Broken Windows' and the Risk of Gonorrhea," *American Journal of Public Health* 90 (2000): 230–36.

47. Benjamin Bailey, "Communication of Respect in Inter-ethnic Service Encounters," *Language in Society* 26, no. 3 (1997): 327–56; P. Devine, "Stereotypes and Prejudice: Automatic and Controlled Components," *Journal of Personality and Social Psychology* 56 (1989): 5–18; Mary L. Inman and Robert S. Baron, "Influence of Prototypes on Perception of Prejudice," *Journal of Personality and Social Psychology* 70, no. 4 (1996): 727–39.

48. Request for applications from National Institutes of Health, "Health Disparities: Linking Biological and Behavioral Determinants: NIH," receipt dated April 26, 2000, http://web.fie.com/htdoc/fed/nih/gen/any/proc/any/11059906.htm.

49. Nancy Krieger and Stephen S. Sidney, "Racial Discrimination and Blood Pressure: The CAR-DIA Study of Young Black and White Adults," *American Journal of Public Health* 86 (1996): 1370–78.

50. David Brown, "Study: Discrimination May Cause Hypertension in Blacks," *Washington Post*, October 24, 1996.

51. National Public Radio, *Morning Edition*, October 24, 1996.

52. Council of Economic Advisers for the President's Initiative on Race, *Changing America: Indicators of Social and Economic Well-being by Race and Hispanic Origin* (Atlanta: Centers for Disease Control, 1998), 41.

53. Brent Staples, "Death by Discrimination? Of Prejudice and Heart Attacks," *New York Times*, November 24, 1996.

54. Brent Staples, "When the Paranoids Turn Out to Be Right," *New York Times*, May 2, 1999.

55. Bruce S. McEwen, "Protective and Damaging Effects of Stress Mediators," *New England Journal of Medicine* 338, no. 3 (1998): 171–79.

56. Harold P. Freeman and Richard Payne, "Racial Inequities in Health Care," *New England Journal of Medicine* 342, no. 14 (2000): 1045–47.

57. Krieger and Sidney, "Racial Discrimination and Blood Pressure," 1375.

58. National Institutes of Health, "Educational Level and Five-Year All-Cause Mortality in the Hypertension Detection and Follow-up Program" (HDFP Cooperative Group), *Hypertension* 9, no. 6 (1987): 641–46.

59. National Heart, Lung and Blood Institute, "NHLBI Study Shows Large Blood Pressure Benefit from Reduced Dietary Sodium" (press release), May 17, 2000.

60. D. D. Savage, L. O. Watkins, C. E. Grim, and S. K. Kumanyika, "Hypertension in Black Populations," in *Hypertension: Pathophysiology, Diagnosis and Management*, edited by J. H. Laragh and B. M. Brenner (New York: Raven Press, 1990), 1837–52. Also note that African Americans, on average, have greater vessel reactivity than whites, and also lower levels of a kidney enzyme called renin that helps regulate blood pressure; see L. L. Watkins, J. E. Dimsdale, and M. G. Ziegler, "Reduced Beta–2-Receptor Mediated Vasodilation in African Americans," *Life Sciences* 57, no. 15 (1995): 1411–16; N. B. Anderson, M. McNeilly, and H. Myers, "Toward Understanding Race Difference in Autonomic Reactivity," in *Individual Differences in Cardiovascular Response to Stress*, edited by J. R. Turner et al. (New York: Plenum Press, 1992), 125–45; Richard P. Lifton, "Molecular Genetics of Human Blood Pressure Variation," *Science* 272 (1996): 676–80.

61. Kawachi, Kennedy, and Wilkinson, *The Society and Population Health Reader*, xvi.

62. James P. Smith and Raynard S. Kingston, "Race, Socioeconomic Status and Health in Late Life," in *Racial and Ethnic Difference in the Health of Older Americans*, edited by Linda G. Martin and Beth J. Soldo (Washington, DC: National Academy Press, 1997), 106–62.

63. Jack M. Guralnick, Kenneth C. Land, Dan Blazer, et al., "Educational Status and Active Life Expectancy Among Older Blacks and Whites," *New England Journal of Medicine* 329 (1993): 110–16.

64. Nancy Moss, "The Body Politic and the Power of Socioeconomic Status," *American Journal of Public Health* 87, no. 9 (September 1997): 1411–12.

65. Centers for Disease Control, "Asthma Mortality and Hospitalization Among Children and Young Adults 1980–1993," *Morbidity and Mortality Weekly Report* 45, no. 17 (1996): 350–53.

66. D. L. Rosenstreich, P. Eggleston, M. Kattan, et al., "The Role of Cockroach Allergy and the Exposure to Cockroach Allergen in Causing Morbidity Among Inner-City Children with Asthma," *New England Journal of Medicine* 336 (1997): 1356–63.

67. *Briefing Note: Employer-Sponsored Health Insurance: Implications for Minority Workers* (New York: Commonwealth Fund, February 1999); see also UCLA Center for Health Policy and Research and Henry J. Kaiser Family Foundation, "Ethnic and Racial Disparities in Access to Health Insurance and Health Care" (August 2000).

68. Marion Ein Lewin and Stewart Altman, eds., *America's Health Care Safety Net: Intact but Endangered* (Washington, DC: Institute of Medicine/National Academy of Sciences Press, 2000).

69. John Z. Ayanian, Betsy A. Kohler, Toshi Abe, and Arnold Epstein, "The Relation Between Health Insurance Coverage and Clinical Outcomes Among Women with Breast Cancer," *New England Journal of Medicine* 329 (1993): 326–31.

70. Bruce G. Link and Jo C. Phelan, "Understanding Sociodemographic Differences in Health: The Role of Fundamental Social Causes," *American Journal of Public Health* 86, no. 4 (1996): 471–73.

71. R. A. Hummer, R. G. Rogers, C. B. Nam, and C. G. Ellison, "Religious Involvement and U.S. Adult Mortality," *Demography* 36 (1999): 273–85; D. Oman and D. Reed, "Religion and Mortality Among Community-Dwelling Elderly," *American Journal of Public Health* 88 (1998): 1469–75.

72. Janice E. Williams, Catherine C. Paton, Ilene C. Seigler, et al., "Anger Proneness Predicts Coronary Heart Disease Risk: Prospective Analysis from the Atherosclerosis Risk in Communities Study," *Circulation* 101 (2000): 2034–39; C. Iribarren, S. Sidney, D. E. Bild, et al., "Association of Hostility with Coronary Artery Calcification in Young Adults," *Journal of the American Medical Association* 283 (2000): 2546–51.

73. Aron Wolfe Siegman, "Cardiovascular Consequences of Expressing and Repressing Anger," in *Anger, Hostility and the Heart,* edited by Aron Wolfe Siegman and Timothy W. Smith (Hillsdale, NJ: Lawrence Erlbaum, 1994), 173–97.

74. S. Leonard Syme, personal communication with the author, October 25, 1999.

75. S. Leonard Syme and Jennifer L. Balfour, "Social Determinants of Disease," in *Public Health and Preventive Medicine,* 14th ed., edited by Robert B. Wallace (New York: McGraw-Hill, 1998), 795–810.

76. John W. Lynch and George A. Kaplan, "Understanding How Inequality in the Distribution of Income Affects Health," in Kawachi, Kennedy, and Wilkinson, *The Society and Population Health Reader,* 202–21.

77. Wilkinson, "Income Distribution and Life Expectancy," 168.

78. Bruce S. McEwen, "Stress, Adaptation and Disease: Allostasis and Allostatic Load," *Annals of the New York Academy of Sciences* 840 (1998): 33–44.

79. S. A. Eversin, D. E. Goldberg, G. A. Kaplan, et al., "Anger Expression and Incident Hypertension," *Psychosomatic Medicine* 60, no. 6 (1998): 730–35; S. B. Miller, L. Dolgoy, M. Friese, and A. Sita, "Dimensions of Hostility and Cardiovascular Response to Interpreted Stress," *Journal of Psychosomatic Research* 41, no. 1 (1996): 91–95.

80. Richard Estrada, "Racism Among Hispanics," *Washington Post,* October 5, 1999.

81. National Center for Health Statistics, *National Vital Statistics Report* 47, no. 10 (November 19, 1998).

82. J. E. Becerra, C. J. Hogue, H. K. Atrash, and N. Perez, "Infant Mortality Among Hispanics: A Portrait of Heterogeneity," *Journal of the American Medical Association* 265 (1991): 217–21.

83. K. S. Markides and J. Coreil, "The Health of Hispanics in the Southwestern United States: An Epidemiologic Paradox," *Public Health Reports* 101, no. 3 (1986): 253–65.

84. S. Guendelman and B. Abrams, "Dietary Intake Among Mexican American Women: Differences and a Comparison with White Non-Hispanic Women," *American Journal of Public Health* 85 (1995): 20–25; W. A. Vega, B. Kolody, J. Hwang, and A. Noble, "Prevalence and Magnitude of Perinatal Substance Exposures in California," *New England Journal of Medicine* 329 (1993): 850–54.

85. Javier I. Escobar, "Immigration and Mental Health: Why Are Immigrants Better Off?" *Archives of General Psychiatry* 55 (1998): 781–82, 782.

86. David E. Hayes-Bautista, "The Secret of L.A.'s Public Health," *Los Angeles Times,* August 6, 2000.

87. R. J. Davis and J. W. Collins Jr., "Bad Outcomes in Black Babies: Race or Racism?" *Ethnicity and Disease* 1 (1991): 236–44, 239.

88. Sharon Schwartz and Kenneth Carpenter, "The Right Answer for the Wrong Question: Consequences of a Type III Error for Public Health Questions," *American Journal of Public Health* 89 (1999): 1175–80; Leslie Berger, "Racial Gap in Infant Deaths and a Search for Reasons," *New York Times,* June 25, 2000.

89. Sheryl Gay Stolberg, "Cultural Issues Pose Obstacles in Cancer Fight," *New York Times,* March 14, 1998.

90. Centers for Disease Control and Prevention, "The National Breast and Cervical Cancer Detection Program: At a Glance, 1999," www.cdc.gov/cancer; S. S. Rajaram and A. Rashidi, "Minority Women and Breast Cancer Screening: The Role of Cultural Explanatory Models," *Preventive Medicine* 27, no. 5, pt. 1 (1998): 757–64.

91. Anthony Valdini and Lucia Cargill, "Access and Barriers to Mammography in New England Community Centers," *Journal of Family Practice* 45, no. 3 (1997): 243–49.

92. L. Song and R. Fletcher, "Breast Cancer Re-screening in Low-Income Women," *American Journal of Preventive Medicine* 15, no. 2 (1998): 128–33; S. W. Chang, K. Kerlikowske, A. Napales-Springer, et al., "Racial Differences in Timelines of Follow-up After Abnormal Screening Mammogram," *Cancer* 78, no. 7 (1996): 1395–1402.

93. Alfred D. Marcus, Celia P. Kaplan, Lori A. Crane, et al., "Reducing Loss-to-Follow-up Among Women with Abnormal Pap Smears," *Medical Care* 36, no. 3 (1998): 397–410.

94. Stolberg, "Cultural Issues Pose Obstacles in Cancer Fight."

95. L. Lacey, J. Whitfeld, W. DeWhite, et al., "Referral Adherence in Inner-City Breast and Cervical Cancer Screening Programs," *Cancer* 72, no. 3 (1993): 950–55.

96. S. H. Kang, J. R. Bloom, and P. S. Romano, "Cancer Screening Among African American Women: The Use of Tests and Social Supports," *American Journal of Public Health* 84, no. 1 (1994): 101–3.

97. "Office of Minority Health: Facing the Challenge," *Urban Health Report* (Fall 1996): 7–10.

98. S. Underwood, "African American Males: Perceptual Determinants of Early Cancer Detection and Cancer Risk Reduction," *Cancer Nursing* 14 (1991): 281–88; K. R. Barber, R. Shaw, M. Folts, et al., "Differences Between African American and Caucasian Men Participating in a Community-Based Prostate Cancer Screening Program," *Journal of Community Health* 23, no. 6 (1998): 441–51.

99. I. J. Powell, K. Schwartz, and M. Hussain, "Removal of the Financial Barrier to Health Care: Does It Impact on Prostate Cancer and Presentation and Survival?: A Comparative Study Between Black and White Men in a Veterans Affairs System," *Urology* 46 (1995): 825.

100. D. G. Sienko, R. A. Hahn, E. M. Mills, et al., "Mammography Use and Outcomes in a Community: The Greater Lansing Area Mammography Study," *Cancer* 71 (1993): 1801–9; N. Breen and L. Kessler, "Changes in the Use of Screening Mammography: Evidence from the 1987 and 1990 National Health Interview Surveys," *American Journal of Public Health* 84 (1994): 62–67; *Breast and Cervical Cancer Screening: Barriers and Use Among Specific Populations,* supp. 3 (Denver: AMC Cancer Research Center, January 1995).

101. V. M. Taylor, B. Thompson, D. E. Montano, et al., "Mammography Use Among Women Attending an Inner-City Clinic," *Journal of Cancer Education* 13, no. 2 (Summer 1998): 96–101.

102. Lorna G. Canlas, "Issues of Health Care Mistrust in East Harlem," *Mount Sinai Journal of Medicine* 66, no. 4 (1999): 257–58. Fatalistic attitudes toward the value of preventive care and the outcomes of disease as well as magical thinking (for example, that the devil can cause cancer, or that mammography machines cause breast cancer) and the use of folk remedies are more prevalent in minority groups; see B. D. Powe, "Fatalism Among Elderly African Americans: Effects on Colorectal Cancer Screening," *Cancer Nursing* 18, no. 5 (1995): 385–92; C. Maynard, L. D. Fisher, E. R. Passamani, and T. Pullum, "Blacks in the Coronary Artery Surgery Study: Race and Clinical Decision Making," *American Journal of Public Health* 76, no. 12 (1986): 1446–48; P. A. Johnson, T. H. Lee, E. F. Cook, et al., "Effect of Race on the Presentation and Management of Patients with Acute Chest Pain," *Annals of Internal Medicine* 118 (1993): 593–601; D. R. Lannin, H. F. Mathews, J. Mitchell, et al., "Influence of Socioeconomic and Cultural Factors on Racial Differences in Late-Stage Presentation of Breast Cancer," *Journal of the American Medical Association* 279, no. 22 (1998): 1801–7; Taylor, Thompson, Montano, et al., "Mammography Use Among Women Attending an Inner-City Clinic."

103. Jennifer S. Haas, J. Steven Udvarhelyi, Carl N. Morris, and Arnold M. Epstein, "The Effect of Providing Health Coverage to Poor Uninsured Pregnant Women in Massachusetts," *Journal of the American Medical Association* 269, no. 1 (1993): 87–91.

104. J. M. Piper, E. F. Mitchel Jr., and W. A. Ray, "Expanded Medicaid Coverage for Pregnant Women to 100 Percent of the Poverty Level," *American Journal of Preventive Medicine* 10, no. 2 (1994): 97–102; L. C. Dubay, G. M. Kenney, S. A. Norton, and B. C. Cohen, "Local Responses to Expanded Medicaid Coverage for Pregnant Women," *Milbank Quarterly* 73, no. 4 (1995): 535–63; M. L. Blankson, R. L. Goldenberg, and B. Keith, "Noncompliance of High-Risk Pregnant Women in Keeping Appointments at an Obstetric Complications Clinic," *Southern Medical Journal* 87, no. 6 (1994): 634–38; M. D. Kogan, M. Kotelchuk, and S. Johnson, "Racial Differences in Late Prenatal Care Visits," *Journal of Perinatology* 13, no. 1 (1993): 14–21; T. A. LaVeist, V. M. Keith, and M. L. Gutierrez, "Black/White Differences in Prenatal Care Utilization: An Assessment of Predisposing and Enabling Factors," *Health Services Research* 30, no. 1 (1995): 43–58.

105. Robert Goldberg, *The Vaccines for Children Programs: A Critique* (Washington, DC: American Enterprise Institute, 1995); Steve Sepe, "Lifesaving Vaccines Underused by Minority Adults," *Closing the Gap: A Newsletter of the Office of Minority Health* [U.S. Department of Health and Human Services] (November 1998): 4.

106. P. E. Cothran and M. Fedor, "African-Americans' Participation in AIDS Research," *International Conference on AIDS* 8, no. 2, D412, abstract PoD 5153; P. A. Simon, F. J. Sorvillo, and R. K. Lapin, "Racial Differences in the Use of Drug Therapy for HIV," *New England Journal of Medicine* 331 (1994): 333–34.

107. Carey Goldberg, "Boston Battles Cancer with a Citywide Mailing," *New York Times*, November 2, 1999.

108. Centers for Disease Control, Prevention Research Centers, "Prevention Works" (fact sheets), September 30, 1999, http://www.cdc.gov/prc/pdf/facts_all.pdf.

109. M. V. Williams, R. M. Parker, D. W. Baker, et al., "Inadequate Functional Health Literacy Among Patients at Two Public Hospitals," *Journal of the American Medical Association* 247 (1995): 1677–82.

110. Ann S. O'Malley, "Cancer—Coverage for Poor Women Too," *Washington Post*, February 1, 2000.

111. Statements available at http://www.apha.org/legislative/policy.

112. "Congressional Campaign Finance Reform" (policy statement 8730) and "Opposition to Contra Aid in Nicaragua" (policy statement 8724), *American Journal of Public Health* 78, no. 2 (1988): 205, 202; American Public Health Association, "Statement on the Military Strikes Against Iraq" (press release), December 17, 1998; APHA, "Cessation of Continued Development of Nuclear Weapons" (policy statement 9804), at www.apha.org/science/98policy.pdf. Granted, the Medicaid issue—unlike concerns about the Middle East, campaign financing and welfare—is directly health-related, but in decrying enhanced state control of the program, the APHA remained true to its record of promoting big-government, left-of-center solutions. Then again, perhaps this is not such a surprise: the APHA has among its internal committees both a "Socialist Caucus" and a "Spirit of 1848 Caucus"—the latter name chosen, its leaders say, to commemorate the publication of the Communist Manifesto.

113. Fernando M. Treviño, personal communication with the author, November 19, 1996.

114. Randy Shilts, *And the Band Played On: Politics, People and the AIDS Epidemic*, Stonewall Inn 2000 edition (New York: St. Martin's Press, 1987), xxii.

115. Chandler Burr, "The AIDS Exception: Privacy Versus Public Health," *Atlantic Monthly* (June 1997): 57–67.

116. Don Hoppert of the American Public Health Association, personal communication with the author, April 10, 2000.

117. Katherine Marconi, "Concentrate on Health, Pursue Politics Judiciously" (letter to the editor), *Nation's Health* (April 1996): 2.

Chapter 2

1. David Foster and Arlene Levinson, "Suicide on a Railroad Track Ends a Celebrity Stalker's Inner Agony," Associated Press, October 6, 1998.

2. Frank Bruni, "Behind the Jokes, a Life of Pain and Delusion," *New York Times*, November 22, 1998.

3. E. Fuller Torrey, "Psychiatric Survivors and Nonsurvivors," *Psychiatric Services* 48, no. 2 (1997): 143. See also Nancy C. Andreasen, "Clients, Consumers, Providers, and Products: Where Will It End?" *American Journal of Psychiatry* 152, no. 8 (1995): 1107–9.

4. Center for Mental Health Services, Substance Abuse and Mental Health Services Administration, "Consumers and Psychiatric–Mental Health Nurses in Dialogue," conference held in Washington, DC, July 26–27, 1999.

5. Coni Kalinowski and Darby Penney, "Empowerment and Women's Health Services," in *Women's Mental Health Services: A Public Health Perspective*, edited by Bruce Lubotsky Levin, Andrea K. Blanch, and Ann Jennings (Thousand Oaks, CA: Sage Publications, 1998), 127–54, 129.

6. Sue Poole, "Where the Dollars Should Go: Voluntary Community Supports," *MadNation*, http://www.madnation.org/tools/needs.htm, accessed April 14, 2000.

7. Jackie Parrish, "CMHS Supports Principles of Empowerment and Self-Help," *National Empowerment Center Newsletter* 1, no. 1 (1994): 2,9.

8. Darby Penney, remarks during "Listening to Us '98," a conference sponsored by the Office of Mental Health Recipient Advisory Committee, Albany, NY, May 28–28, 1998; see also http://www.omh.state.ny.us/qvol4no2.htm.

9. "Is the Demonization of People Diagnosed with Mental Illness a Hate Crime?" *Mad Nation*, http://www.madnation.org/news/IOC/hate.htm, accessed November 26, 1999.

10. Chris Lydgate, "The Guinea Pigs' Rebellion," *Willamette Week*, September 1, 1999.

11. Scott Snedecor, "The Death of Mental Illness," *National Empowerment Center Newsletter* 3, no. 3 (1994): 6–7.

12. Pat Deegan, "The Recovery/Healing/Empowerment Project," *National Empowerment Newsletter* 1, no. 1 (1994): 4.

13. Paolo Del Vecchio, personal communication with the author, December 22, 1998.

14. National Mental Health Consumers' Self-Help Clearinghouse, "National Summit of Mental Health Consumers and Survivors," www.mhselfhelp.org/summit.html, accessed March 31, 2000.

15. Lydgate, "The Guinea Pigs' Rebellion."

16. David Oaks, "Tubman Project," Support Coalition International list serve, dendron@efn.org, September 2, 1999.

17. "Huge Victory in Oregon: We Helped Stop Oregon's Attorney General Bill," Support Coalition International list serve, dendron@efn.org, May 6, 1999.

18. Niyyah, "Addressing Women's Mental Health," *Consumer Affairs Bulletin of the Center for Mental Health Services* 3, no. 2 (1998): 2–3. Duplicating many of her comments under the pseudonym Niyyah in the *Consumer Affairs Bulletin*, McKinney gave the keynote address at the Maine Department of Mental Health Office of Trauma Services conference, Portland, October 18–20, 1998.

19. National Disability Council, "From Privileges to Rights: People Labeled with Psychiatric Disabilities Speak for Themselves," www.ncd.gov/newsroom/publications/privileges.html, accessed April 2, 2000.

20. Marca Bristo (chairperson of the National Council on Disabilities), letter of transmittal to the president, January 20, 2000, www.ncd.gov/newsroom/publications/privileges.html.

21. Al Siebert, "Successful Schizophrenia—The Survivor Personality," paper presented at Alternatives '95, St. Paul, Minnesota, August 3–5, 1995.

22. Paolo del Vecchio, list-serve announcement about Alternatives '99, September 24, 1999, http://alternatives.contac.org.

23. In an opinion piece, Zinman called the event a "controlled infomercial"; see Sally Zinman, "Band-Aids for the Mind," *San Jose Mercury News*, June 20, 1999.

24. Jeffrey L. Geller, Julie-Marie Brown, William H. Fisher, et al., "A National Survey of 'Consumer Empowerment' at the State Level," *Psychiatric Services* 49, no. 4 (1998): 498–503.

25. Jeffrey Geller, M.D., personal communication with the author, November 6, 1998.

26. Center for Mental Health Services, Substance Abuse and Mental Health Services Administration, "Responding to the Behavioral Healthcare Issues of Persons with Histories of Physical and Sexual Abuse, July 1998" (national trauma experts' meeting), Alexandria, VA, April 2–3, 1998, 14.

27. Rodney E. Copeland, "Vermont's Vision of a Public System for Developmental and Mental Health Services Without Coercion," Vermont Department of Developmental and Mental Health Services, http://www.state.vt.us/dmh/rod.pdf, accessed January 18, 2000.

28. Andrea Sheerin, personal communication with the author, January 14, 1999.

29. Laura Van Tosh and Paolo Del Vecchio, *Consumer-Survivor Operated Self-Help Programs: A Technical Report* (Washington, DC: U.S. Department of Health and Human Services, January 1998), 1–20.

30. Public Health Service Block Grants (1998), Public Law 102-321, Title 42, Chapter 6A.

31. Center for Mental Health Services, "Center for Mental Health Services Names Consumer/Survivor Subcommittee to Work with Advisory Council" (press release), August 3, 2000.

32. Paul F. Stavis, personal communication with the author, January 6, 1999.

33. Center for Mental Health Services, U.S. Department of Health and Human Services, *Consumer Affairs Bulletin* 4, no. 1 (Spring 1999); see http://www.cstprogram.org.

34. Information provided by National Technical Assistance Center for State Mental Health Planning, Alexandria, VA, January 14, 1999.

35. E. Fuller Torrey, personal communication with the author, February 24, 2000.

36. Bernard Zuber, personal communication with the author, July 21, 1999.

37. Moe Armstrong, personal communication with the author, December 3, 1998.

38. Robert E. Nikkel, Garrett Smith, and David Edwards, "A Consumer-Oriented Case Management Project," *Psychiatric Services* 43, no. 6 (1992): 577–79.

39. Daniel B. Fisher, "Health Care Reform Based on an Empowerment Model of Recovery by People with Psychiatric Disabilities," *Hospital and Community Psychiatry* 45, no. 9 (1994): 913.

40. Sally L. Satel, "The Madness of Deinstitutionalization," *Wall Street Journal*, February 20, 1996.

41. Dan Morain and Julie Marquis, "Leaving State Hospitals Sent Many into Psychotic Abyss," *Los Angeles Times*, November 22, 1999.

42. D. J. Jaffe, personal communication with the author, December 16, 1998.

43. Rael Jean Isaac and Virginia C. Armat, *Madness in the Streets: How Psychiatry and the Law Abandoned the Mentally Ill* (New York: Free Press, 1990), 250. Judge Lippman was overruled when the city appealed. Brown remained hospitalized but refused medication. An evaluation by an independent psychiatrist resulted in the recommendation that she not be medicated against her will. At that point Bellevue decided to release her, since there was no point in retaining a patient who could not be treated (256–60).

44. Rick Hampson, "An Icon of Homelessness Nestled in Oblivion" (Associated Press), *Bergen Record*, June 9, 1991.

45. Associated Press, "Hospitalization Foe Is Back in Bellevue," *New York Times*, August 26, 1993.

46. Norman Siegel, personal communication with the author, March 30, 2000.

47. Hampson, "An Icon of Homelessness Nestled in Oblivion."

48. Isaac and Armat, *Madness in the Streets*, 58.

49. Ron Honberg, J.D., personal communication with the author, January 6, 1996; Rael Jean Isaac, "Protect the Mentally Ill from Their Advocates," *Wall Street Journal*, May 7, 1991.

50. Max Fink, *Electroshock: Restoring the Mind* (Oxford: Oxford University Press, 1999), 95–97.

51. Michael Lesser, M.D. (medical director of the New York State Department of Mental Health, Mental Retardation and Alcoholism Services), personal communication with the author, November 3, 1998; James L. Curtis, M.D. (chairman of psychiatry, Harlem Hospital), personal communication with the author, October 22, 1998.

52. Erica Goode, "Federal Report Praising Electroshock Stirs Uproar," *New York Times,* October 6, 1999.

53. David Oaks, Support Coalition International list serve, dendron@efn.org, September 24, 1999.

54. Vermont Protection and Advocacy (Montpelier), memo, January 3, 2000.

55. Mary Zdanowicz (executive director of the Treatment Advocacy Center, Arlington, VA) and Carla Jacobs (NAMI board member), personal communications with the author, both on April 5, 2000.

56. Isaac and Armat, *Madness in the Streets,* 269.

57. APA President Jerry Weiner, letter to CMHS Director Bernard S. Arons, February 13, 1995.

58. Elaine Sutton Mbionwu, "Involuntary Outpatient Commitment: If It Isn't Voluntary . . . Maybe It Isn't Treatment," *Protection and Advocacy Systems News* 4, no. 5 (Winter 1999): 1–2.

59. NAMI, press release, October 14, 1998.

60. Sylvia Caras, "The Downside of the Family-Organized Mental Illness Advocacy Movement," *Psychiatric Services* 49, no. 6 (1998): 763–64.

61. Douglas Smith (Anti-Psychiatry Coalition), letter to Thomas Finneran (speaker of the Massachusetts legislature), July 2, 1998; posted at www.antipsychiatry.org, accessed April 16, 2000.

62. For a description of the mental health court in King County, Washington, see http://www.metrokc.gov/kcdc/mhhome.htm, accessed April 2, 2000.

63. Fox Butterfield, "Prisons Replace Hospitals for the Nation's Mentally Ill," *New York Times,* March 5, 1998.

64. Carla Jacobs, personal communication with the author, January 6, 1999.

65. Pat Risser, "Warning: Mental Illness Courts," entry on list serve parisser@att.net, September 10, 1999; see also http://home.att.net/~PatRisser.

66. Judi Chamberlin, entry on list serve parisser@att.net, September 10, 1999.

67. "The Last Minority," panel presentation at the Alternatives '99 conference, Houston, October 22, 1999.

68. "Eve," personal communication with the author, December 4, 1998.

69. Bazelon Center for Mental Health Law, *Annual Report 1993–1994,* 16.

70. Henry Korman, Diane Engster, and Bonnie M. Milstein, "Housing as a Tool of Coercion," in *Coercion and Aggressive Community Treatment,* edited by Deborah L. Dennis and John Monahan (New York: Plenum Press, 1996), 110–11.

71. "Group Home Controls Sought: Clifton Backed by State League," *Bergen County Record,* October 27, 1998; "Clifton Home Must Change Staff, Clients," *Bergen County Record,* November 22, 1998.

72. National Mental Health Association, "Study Contradicts Cultural Image of Violent Mentally Ill" (press release), May 14, 1998.

73. Larry Sosowsky, "Explaining the Increased Arrest Rate Among Mental Patients: A Cautionary Note," *American Journal of Psychiatry* 137, no. 12 (1980): 1602–5.

74. M. Eronen, J. Tiihonen, P. Hakola, et al., "Schizophrenia and Homicidal Behavior," *Schizophrenia Bulletin* 22, no. 1 (1996): 83–89.

75. John M. Dawson and Patrick Langan, *Special Report: Murder in Families* (Washington, DC: Bureau of Justice Statistics, U.S. Department of Justice, 1994).

76. John Monahan, "Mental Disorder and Violent Behavior," *American Psychologist* 47 (1992): 511–21.

77. Sally Satel and D. J. Jaffe, "Violent Fantasies," *National Review,* July 20, 1998: 37.

78. Jonathan Stanley, comments on outpatient commitment at a press conference held by the attorney general of New York State, January 28, 1999.

79. William Gardner, Charles W. Lidz, Steven K. Hoge, et al., "Patients' Revision of Their Beliefs About the Need for Hospitalization," *American Journal of Psychiatry* 156 (1999): 1385–91.

80. Ibid.

81. Paul S. Applebaum, "Outpatient Commitment: The Problems and the Promise," *American Journal of Psychiatry* 143, no. 10 (1986): 1270–72.

82. Policy Research Associates, "Research Study of the New York City Involuntary Outpatient Commitment Pilot Program," prepared for the New York City Department of Mental Health, Mental Retardation and Alcoholism Services, December 4, 1998.

83. The Support Coalition produces an antipsychiatry newspaper called *Dendron* that promotes the "Heal Normality, Naturally" campaign, warning patients about the dire consequences of psychiatric medications and electroconvulsive therapy.

84. Carla Cubit (Support Coalition member), testimony at the Bellevue hearing, December 16, 1998.

85. Howard Telson, M.D., personal communication with the author, December 17, 1998.

86. Xavier Amador, personal communication with the author, December 20, 1999.

87. Michael Winerip, "Man Who Pushed Woman onto Tracks Needed Supervision, Report Said," *New York Times*, November 5, 1999.

88. Raymond Hernandez, "Pataki Proposes Curb on Releases for Mentally Ill," *New York Times*, November 10, 1999.

89. Center for the Community Interest, "The Strange Politics of Outpatient Commitment," *CCI Friday Fax* (weekly newsletter), June 11, 1999; www.comunityinterest.org, accessed April 2, 2000.

90. Mental Patients Liberation Alliance, testimony at the Bellevue hearing, December 16, 1998; see also New York Association of Psychiatric Rehabilitation Services, testimony at the Bellevue hearing, December 16, 1998.

91. See, for example, Eric M. Weiss, "Deadly Restraint: A Nationwide Pattern of Death," *Hartford Courant*, October 11, 1998.

Chapter 3

1. Questionable Nursing Practices Task Force, National Council for Reliable Health Information (New York), personal communication with the author, March 10, 1999.

2. Lynda Juall Carpenito, *Nursing Diagnosis: Application to Clinical Practice*, 6th ed. (Philadelphia: Lippincott, 1995), 355–58.

3. Cynthia Poznanski Hutchison, "Healing Touch," *American Journal of Nursing* 99, no. 4 (1999): 43–48, 48.

4. Rebecca Witmer, "Hands That Heal: The Art of Therapeutic Touch," at www.dcn.davis.-ca.us/go/btcarrol/skeptic/tt.html.

5. Nurse Healers–Professional Associates International, www.therapeutic-touch.org/html/touch.-html, accessed April 9, 2000. In Canada, the College of Nurses of Ontario 1990 Implementation Standards incorporated TT, as documented in Witmer, "Hands That Heal."

6. Described in Sharon Fish, "Therapeutic Touch: Healing Science or Psychic Midwife?" *Christian Research Journal* (Summer 1995): 28–38; as advertised in *The American Nurse* (newsletter of the American Nurses Association), convention bulletin insert, January 1994.

7. Colorado State Board of Nursing, *Subcommittee to Investigate the Awarding of Continuing Education Units to Nurses for the Study of Therapeutic Touch and Other Nontraditional and Complementary Healing Modalities: Recommendations* (Denver: Colorado State Board of Nursing, 1992); available on Rocky Mountain Skeptics web site, http://www.bcn.boulder.co.us/community/rms/rms-tt3.html.

8. Barbara Ehrenreich and Deirdre English, *Witches, Midwives and Nurses: A History of Women Healers* (New York: Feminist Press at the City University of New York, 1973).

9. Linda Rosa, Emily Rosa, Larry Sarner, and Stephen Barrett, "A Close Look at Therapeutic Touch," *Journal of the American Medical Association* 279 (1998): 1005–10.

10. Susan B. Collins, letter to the editor, *Journal of the American Medical Association* 280, no. 22 (1998): 1905.

11. Mary Ireland, letter to the editor, *Journal of the American Medical Association* 280, no. 22 (1998): 1906.

12. Terence Monmaney and Louis Sahagun, "Fourth Grader's Study Rebuts Touch Therapy," *Los Angeles Times*, April 1, 1998.

13. Nurse Healers–Professional Associates International, http://www.therapeutic-touch.org/html/responses_to_jama.html.

14. Andrew Weil, "Ask Dr. Weil," http://pathfinder.com/drweil, accessed December 1998.

15. Carpenito, *Nursing Diagnosis*, 356.

16. The National Council for Reliable Health Information is part of the National Council Against Health Fraud; see www.ncahf.org.

17. Donal P. O'Mathuna, "Representation of Original Research in Therapeutic Touch Reviews," forthcoming in *Image: Journal of Nursing Scholarship*.

18. Dolores Krieger, *Accepting Your Power to Heal: The Personal Practice of Therapeutic Touch* (Santa Fe, NM: Bear and Co., 1993), 3–4.

19. James Randi, personal communication with the author, February 17, 2000; see James Randi's web site for information on how to apply for the $1 million Paranormal Challenge: www.randi.org/research/challenge/index.html.

20. Wallace Sampson, M.D., personal communication with the author, March 20, 2000.

21. Robert Park, *Voodoo Science: The Road from Foolishness to Fraud* (New York: Oxford University Press, 2000), 67.

22. Stephen E. Straus, "New Center Director States Complementary Agenda," *Journal of the American Medical Association* 283, no. 8 (2000): 990–91.

23. Melvin Konner, review of *Afterwards, You're a Genius* by Chip Brown, *New York Times Book Review*, April 11, 1999.

24. Wallace L. Sampson, M.D., "'Alternative Medicine': A Description of the 'Alternative Medicine' Movement, and a Survey of Education at U.S. Medical Schools," forthcoming in *Academic Press*.

25. "Tang Center Gets $5 Million," *Legacy* [University of Chicago] (Winter 1999–2000): 1.

26. Jay Greene, "Anesthesia Turf War Heats up in a Battle over Supervision," *American Medical Association News* 42, no. 10 (1999): 1.

27. Jo Ann Ashley, "Power Is Structured Misogyny: Implications for the Politics of Care," *Advances in Nursing Science* 2, no. 3 (1980): 3–22.

28. Ehrenreich and English, *Witches, Midwives and Nurses*, 43; Susan H. Cummings, "Attila the Hun Versus Attila the Hen: Gender Socialization of the American Nurse," *Nursing Administration Quarterly* 19, no. 2 (1995): 19–25.

29. Adeline R. Falk Rafael (American Nurses Association), http://www.ana.org/ojin/letters/-t1c1.htm, accessed April 8, 1999.

30. Adeline R. Falk Raphael, "Power and Caring: A Dialectic in Nursing," *Advances in Nursing Science* 19, no. 1 (1996): 3–17.

31. A. J. Baumgart, "The Quality of Work Life of Hospital Nurses: The Legacy of History," in *Women in Women's Work: An Exploratory Study of Nurses' Perspectives of Quality Work Environments*, edited by C. Attridge and M. Callahan (Victoria, BC: University of Victoria, 1987).

32. Jean Watson, "Postmodernism and Knowledge Development in Nursing," *Nursing Science Quarterly* 8, no. 2 (Summer 1995): 60–64.

33. P. Hickson and C. A. Holmes, "Nursing the Postmodern Body," *Nursing Inquiry* 1 (1994): 3–14.

34. Sharon McGuire, "Global Migration and Health: Ecofeminist Perspectives," *Advances in Nursing Science* 21, no. 2 (1998): 1–16.

35. S. Ruangjiratain and J. Kendal, "Understanding Women's Risk of HIV Infection in Thailand Through Critical Hermeneutics," *Advances in Nursing Science* 21, no. 2 (1998): 42–51.

36. Michele J. Eliason, "Correlates of Prejudice in Nursing Students," *Journal of Nursing Education* 37, no. 1 (1998): 27–29.

37. John R. Phillips, "Inquiry into the Paranormal," *Nursing Science Quarterly* 9, no. 3 (1996): 89–91.

38. Sarah Glazer, "Postmodern Nursing," *The Public Interest* (Summer 2000): 3–16.

39. As quoted in J. Watson, "New Dimensions of Human Caring Theory," *Nursing Science Quarterly* 1, no. 4 (1988): 175–81.

40. Gail J. Mitchell, "Questioning Evidence-Based Practice for Nursing," *Nursing Science Quarterly* 10, no. 4 (1997): 154–55.

41. Julie Sochalski, personal communication with the author, February 26, 1999.

42. Mark Avis, personal communication with the author, March 24, 1999; see also Mark Avis, "Objectivity in Nursing Research: Observations and Objections," *International Journal of Nursing Studies* 35, no. 3 (1998): 141–45.

43. Lorraine N. Smith, "An Analysis and Reflections on the Quality of Nursing Research in 1992," *Journal of Advanced Nursing* 19, no. 2 (1994): 385–93, 385.

44. Ibid., 387.

45. Susan R. Gortner, "Nursing's Syntax Revisited: A Critique of Philosophies Said to Influence Nursing Theories," *International Journal of Nursing Studies* 30, no. 6 (1993): 477–88.

46. Barbara J. Drew, "Devaluation of Biological Knowledge," *Image: Journal of Nursing Scholarship* 20, no. 1 (1988): 25–27.

47. Donal P. O'Mathuna, personal communication with the author, February 28, 1999.

48. Kevin Courcey, personal communication with the author, March 10, 1999.

49. American Nurses Association, *Code for Nurses with Interpretive Statements,* publication G-56 (Washington, DC: American Nurses Publishing, 1985), 15.

50. Questionable Nursing Practices Task Force, National Council for Reliable Health Information, www.ncrhi.org, accessed April 14, 2000.

51. Elaine E. Bishop, personal communication with the author, March 19, 1999.

52. Sharon Fish, "Therapeutic Touch: Healing Science or Psychic Midwife?" *Christian Research Journal* (Summer 1995): 28–38, 38.

53. Equal Employment Opportunity Commission, "Policy Guidance on 'New Age' Training Programs Which Conflict with Employees' Religious Beliefs," Notice N–915.022, September 2, 1988.

54. Henry N. Claman, "Report of the Chancellor's Committee on Therapeutic Touch," delivered to Chancellor Vincent Fulginiti, M.D., University of Colorado Health Sciences Center, July 6, 1994.

55. Henry N. Claman, M.D., personal communication with the author, March 20, 1999.

56. Gina Kolata, "A Child's Paper Poses a Medical Challenge," *New York Times,* April 1, 1998.

57. http://www.ph.utexas.edu/nursing/ce/ce.html, item from March 9, 1999.

58. Stephen Barnett, M.D., personal communication with the author, March 6, 1999.

59. Roahn H. Wynar, personal communication with the author, March 29, 1999.

60. Minette Marrin, "Nurses Are the Problem," *London Telegraph,* January 10, 1999.

61. Janet Warren and Myles Harris, "Extinguishing the Lamp: The Crisis in Nursing in Digby Anderson," in *Come Back, Miss Nightingale: Trends in Professions Today,* edited by Digby C. Anderson (London: Social Affairs Unit, St. Edmundsbury Press, 1998), 11–36.

62. Ibid.

63. John Clare, "Britain Bottom of Literacy League," *Telegraph,* June 15, 2000.

64. Division of Nursing, Bureau of Health Professions, Health Resources Services Administration, "National Sample Survey of Registered Nurses" (1996).

65. Maryann F. Fralic, personal communication with the author, December 9, 1999.

66. Marge Bradley, letter to the editor, *New Haven Register,* February 17, 1998.

67. Todd S. Purdum, "California to Set Level of Staffing for Nursing Care," *New York Times*, October 12, 1999.

68. Claire M. Fagin, "Nurses, Patients and Managed Care," *New York Times*, March 16, 1999.

69. Peter T. Kilborn, "Registered Nurses in Short Supply at Hospitals Nationwide," *New York Times*, March 23, 1999.

70. P. I. Buerhaus, D. O. Staiger, and D. I. Auerbach, "Implications of an Aging Registered Nurse Workforce," *Journal of the American Medical Association* 283 (2000): 2948–54.

71. Jill Leovy, "Dropout, Failure Rates in Nursing Programs Soar," *Los Angeles Times*, November 23, 1999.

72. Julie Herda, "Nursing Shortage," *Los Angeles Times*, November 28, 1999.

73. National Organization of Nurse Practitioner Faculties, http://www.nonpf.com/culture.htm.

74. Linda Rosa, personal communication with the author, April 12, 1999.

Chapter 4

1. Patricia Ireland, "Statement of National Organization of Women" (press release), October 27, 1999, http://www.now.org/press/10-99/10-27-99.html, accessed April 15, 2000; Breast Cancer Fund, "Call for Research into the Possible Environmental Causes of Breast Cancer," http://www.breastcancerfund.org/advocacy_campaign.html, accessed April 15, 2000; U.S. Rep. Nancy Pelosi, "Pelosi Seeks Research into Environmental Links to Breast Cancer, Other Diseases, October 27, 1999," http://www.house.gov/pelosi/brcancpr.htm, accessed April 15, 2000.

2. Breast Cancer Fund, http://www.breastcancerfund.org/campaign_oped.html, accessed June 22, 2000.

3. National Cancer Institute, "Surveillance Epidemiology and End Results Database," table IV-3, http://seer.cancer.gov/publications/CSR1973_1997/breast.pdf.

4. Stephen H. Safe, "Xenoestrogens and Breast Cancer," *New England Journal of Medicine* 337, no. 18 (1997): 1303–4.

5. Theo Colborn, Dianne Dumanoski, and John Peterson Myers, *Our Stolen Future: Are We Threatening Our Fertility, Intelligence, and Survival?: A Scientific Detective Story* (New York: Dutton, 1996).

6. S. F. Arnold, D. M. Klotz, B. M. Collins, et al., "Synergistic Activation of Estrogen Receptor with Combinations of Environmental Chemicals," *Science* 272 (1996): 1489–92.

7. Safe, "Xenoestrogens and Breast Cancer."

8. Jennifer R. Myhre, "The Breast Cancer Movement: Seeing Beyond Consumer Activism," *Journal of the American Medical Women's Association* 59 (1999): 29–30, 30.

9. Christiane Northrup, *Women's Bodies, Women's Wisdom: Creating Physical and Emotional Health and Healing* (New York: Bantam Books, 1998), 90, 91, 95.

10. Ibid., 90.

11. "Weaving Women's Health Together," distributed at the annual meeting of the Foundation for Women's Health, Washington, DC, April 23–26, 1999.

12. Kelley Phillips, "Beyond the Debate," *American College of Women's Health Physicians News* (March 1999): 2.

13. A. A. Skolnick, "Women's Health Specialty, Other Issues on Agenda of 'Reframing' Conference," *Journal of the American Medical Association* 268 (1992): 1813–14.

14. Ibid.

15. Elena V. Rios and Clay E. Simpson Jr., "Curriculum Enhancement in Medical Education: Teaching Cultural Competence and Women's Health for a Changing Society," *Journal of the American Medical Women's Association*, supp., vol. 53, no. 3 (1998): 114–20.

16. Sue V. Rosser, *Women's Health: Missing from U.S. Medicine* (Bloomington: Indiana University Press, 1994).

17. Cited in Carolyn Newbergh, "The Picture of Women's Health," *Public Health* [University of California at Berkeley School of Public Health] (Spring–Summer 1995): 3.

18. Hillary Rodham Clinton, speech delivered July 19, 1993, excerpted in a brochure of the Society for the Advancement of Women's Health Research.

19. Vice President Al Gore, remarks at a "Women for Gore" event, June 1, 1999; see Gore 2000 web site, http://www.algore2000.com/speeches/speeches_wfg_060199.html.

20. Office of Research on Women's Health, "Implementation of the NIH Guidelines on the Inclusion of Women and Minorities as Subjects in Clinical Research, Comprehensive Report," fiscal year 1997 tracking data (May 2000), http://www4.od.nih.gov/orwh/tracking97.html. Note that women represented 74.8 percent of all phase 3 clinical trials funded in 1997, and 61.9 percent of all extramural research (phase 3 included).

21. Cancer Information Service, National Cancer Institute, 800-422-6237, June 22, 1999.

22. Ed Bartlett, personal communication with the author, June 15, 2000, on a bill to create a men's health office at NIH, proposed by Congressman Randy Cunningham (R-CA).

23. National Cancer Institute, "Surveillance Epidemiology and End Results Database," http://seer.cancer.gov/Publications/CSR1973_1997/prostate.pdf and http://seer.cancer.gov/Publications/CSR1973_1993/breast.pdf.

24. Cary P. Gross, Gerard F. Anderson, and Neil R. Powe, "The Relation Between Funding by the National Institutes of Health and the Burden of Disease," *New England Journal of Medicine* 340, no. 24 (1999): 1881–87.

25. Wirthlin Worldwide, "Myths and Misperceptions About Aging and Women's Health: Initial Findings Prepared for the National Council on the Aging," November 1997.

26. Elaine Ratner, *The Feisty Woman's Breast Cancer Book* (Alameda, CA: Hunter House, 1999), 20, 14.

27. S. L. Murphy, National Center for Health Statistics, "Deaths: Final Data for 1998," *National Vital Statistics Reports* 48, no. 11 (2000).

28. Jane E. Brody, "Personal Health: Coping with Fear: Keeping Breast Cancer in Perspective," *New York Times,* October 12, 1999.

29. As of fall 2000, these bills are still under consideration. The clinical relevance of these bills is hard to dispute. Yet other legislation seems almost frivolous as topics for congressional attention. The Right to Breast-feed Act, for example, is a free-standing bill protecting a woman's right to breast-feed on federal property. The Safe and Effective Breast Pumps Act of 1999 addresses an issue that could have been handled on a regulatory level by the Food and Drug Administration.

30. "NIH Consensus Development Conference on Breast Cancer Screening for Women Ages Forty to Forty-nine," January 21–23, 1997, http://odp.od.nih.gov/consensus/103/103_abstract.pdf.

31. "U.S. Senate to NCI: Return to Old Guidelines, Stop 'Mixed Messages' on Mammograms," *Cancer Letter* 23, no. 6 (1997): 1–5. Note that among the professional groups urging mammograms in the forty-to-forty-nine age group were radiologists. Most other physician groups supported the conference recommendation and suggested that the radiologists had a considerable conflict of interest.

32. Quoted in "NCI Faced Pressure from Congress, HHS, White House on Mammography Statement," *Cancer Letter* 23, no. 14 (1997): 1–6.

33. Quoted in "NCAB Endorses Mammograms for 'Average Risk' Women 40–49; Screening Schedules May Vary Among Individuals," *Cancer Letter* 23, no. 13 (1997): 4–7.

34. Virginia L. Ernster," Mammography Screening for Women Aged 40–49: A Guidelines Saga and a Clarion Call for Informed Decision Making," *American Journal of Public Health* 87 (1997): 1103–6.

35. U.S. Commission on Civil Rights, *The Health Care Challenge: Acknowledging Disparity, Confronting Discrimination, and Ensuring Equality,* vol. 1, *The Role of Governmental and Private Health Care Programs and Initiatives* (September 1999), 85.

36. Ibid., 61.

37. Janet Bickel, "Women in Academic Medicine," *Journal of the American Medical Women's Association* 55 (2000): 10–12.

38. Valerie A. Jones, "Why Aren't There More Women Surgeons?" *Journal of the American Medical Association* 283, no. 5 (2000): 670. Note that women researchers are more likely than their male counterparts to choose an academic career at a small liberal arts college, where the pressure to produce research findings is less intense and there is more sense of personal freedom to start a family. For a review of surveys of young women scientists, see Alison Schneider, "Female Scientists Turn Their Backs on Jobs at Research Universities," *Chronicle of Higher Education* (August 18, 2000): A12–14.

39. "Appendix 2: Graduate Medical Education," *Journal of the American Medical Association* 282, no. 9 (1999): 893. Note that the most popular specialty among both men and women is internal medicine (general medicine), which recruits about one-fifth of all graduating students, according to the Association of American Medical Colleges. About 9 percent of the men choose family practice compared with 13 percent of women.

40. U.S. Commission on Civil Rights, *The Health Care Challenge,* 197.

41. Division of Statistical Analysis, National Institutes of Health, July 12, 1999.

42. Robert F. Moore (Division of Statistical Analysis, NIH), personal communication with the author, July 12, 1999.

43. Lynn Nonnemaker, "Women Physicians in Academic Medicine: New Insights from Cohort Studies," *New England Journal of Medicine* 342 (2000): 399–405.

44. Catherine DeAngelis, "Women in Academic Medicine: New Insights, Same Sad News," *New England Journal of Medicine* 342 (2000): 426–27.

45. Doreen Kimura, letter to National Science and Engineering Research Council, circulated January 4, 2000, on National Association of Scholars list serve.

46. A. D. Irvine, "Jack and Jill and Employment Equity," *Dialogue* 35 (1996): 255–91.

47. D. Lubinski and C. P. Benbow, "Gender Differences in Abilities and Preferences Among the Gifted: Implications for the Math/Science Pipeline," *Current Directions in Psychological Science* 1, no. 2 (1992): 61–66.

48. U.S. Commission on Civil Rights, *The Health Care Challenge,* ix.

49. Ibid., 205. The commission also charges that women have been shortchanged in the distribution of cadaver kidneys (84). Data from the United Network for Organ Sharing, the definitive national registry of transplant data, show that women, as a group, received kidneys from deceased donors as needed. The data confirm that women and men received kidneys from deceased donors in roughly the same proportion as they donated them: in 1997, 40 percent of kidneys in the donor pool came from, and went to, women, and 60 percent came from, and went to, men; see UNOS, "1998 Organ Procurement and Transplantation Network Annual Report," http://www.unos.org/-Data/anrpt98/ar98_table13_03_kid.htm.

50. Olympia Snowe, "Mammograms Save Lives," *Washington Post,* February 11, 1997.

51. Andrew G. Kadar, "The Sex-Bias Myth in Medicine," *Atlantic Monthly* (August 1994): 66–70; Andrew G. Kadar, letter to the editor, *Atlantic Monthly* (November 1994): 17.

52. J. Craig Nelson, M.D. (professor of psychiatry at Yale University School of Medicine), personal communication with the author, February 8, 2000; Paul Leber, M.D. (former FDA division head), personal communication with the author, February 8, 2000.

53. Frederick K. Goodwin, M.D., professor of psychiatry, George Washington University Medical School, personal communication with the author, August 14, 2000.

54. Ely Lilly Co., "Welcome Back: Why Is It Important That We Discuss the Issue of Women and Depression?" (newsletter), 7; Nancy Dickey, M.D. (of the American Medical Association), testimony before House Select Committee on Aging, Housing and Consumer Interests Subcommittee, July 24, 1990.

55. Ruth B. Merkatz, "Women in Clinical Trials of New Drugs: A Change in Food and Drug Administration Policy," *New England Journal of Medicine* 329 (1993): 292–96, 294.

56. Anna C. Mastroianni, Ruth Faden, and Daniel Federman, *Women and Health Research* (Washington, DC: National Academy Press, 1994).

57. Ely Lilly Co., "Welcome Back," 7; *Insights* (newsletter of the Jacobs Institute for Women's Health) 1 (January 1997): 1.

58. Harvard Medical School, *Harvard Women's Health Watch*, promotional letter, received June 6, 2000.

59. NIH Office of Research on Women's Health, "Implementation of the NIH Guidelines on the Inclusion of Women and Minorities as Subjects in Clinical Research," December 1999, http://www4.od.nih.gov/orwh/tracking97.html.

60. Memo to the co-chairs of the National Academy of Sciences and the Institute of Medicine Committee on the legal and ethical issues relating to the inclusion of women in clinical studies, reprinted in Mastroianni, Faden, and Federman, *Women and Health Research*, 224 (appendix A).

61. David J. Morrow, "Women's Drugs: Big in Profits, Narrow in Scope," *New York Times*, June 13, 1999.

62. Don Luckit (NIH Office of AIDS Research), personal communication with the author, June 22, 1999.

63. National Heart, Lung and Blood Institute Advisory Council, "Women's Health Issues," presentation at the 159th NHLBI meeting, Bethesda, MD, September 6, 1990, 14. Note that the NIH-funded Baltimore Longitudinal Study of Aging began in 1958 but did not enroll women until 1978. I have not been able to discern any clinical or logistical justification for excluding women for the first twenty years of the study, which is still ongoing.

64. J. H. Gurwitz, N. F. Col, and J. Avorn, "The Exclusion of the Elderly and Women from Clinical Trials in Acute Myocardial Infarction," *Journal of the American Medical Association* 268 (1992): 1417–22.

65. Steering Committee of the Physician Health Study Research Group, "The Final Report of the Aspirin Component of the Ongoing Physician Health Study," *New England Journal of Medicine* 321 (1989): 129–35. The article notes a high rate of compliance. "By January 25, 1988, the participants had been followed for an average of 60.2 months; 99.7% were still providing information on morbidity, and the vital status of all 22,071 doctors was known."

66. National Heart, Lung and Blood Institute Advisory Council, "Women's Health Issues," 9.

67. U. E. Heidland, M. P. Heintzen, W. J. Klimek, et al., "Acute Complications and Restenosis in Women Undergoing Percutaneous Transluminal Coronary Angioplasty: Is It Possible to Define Sex Differences and to Determine Risk Factors?" *Journal of Cardiovascular Risk* 5, nos. 5–6 (1998): 297–302; S. F. Kelsey, M. James, A. L. Holubkov, et al., "Results of Percutaneous Transluminal Coronary Angioplasty in Women: 1985–1986 National Heart, Lung and Blood Institute's Coronary Angioplasty Registry," *Circulation* 87 (1993): 720–27.

68. Michael E. DeBakey, M.D., personal communication with the author, December 8, 1999.

69. Stephen Colvin, letter to the editor, *Wall Street Journal*, May 24, 1999.

70. D. B. Mark and D. B. Pryor, "Screening and Diagnostic Testing in Women with Suspected Coronary Artery Disease," in *Cardiovascular Health and Disease in Women*, edited by Nanette K. Wenger (Greenwich, CT: Le Jacq Communications, 1993), 81–90.

71. J. H. Gurwitz, T. J. McLaughlin, D. J. Willison, et al., "Delayed Hospital Presentation in Patients Who Have Had Acute Myocardial Infarction," *Annals of Internal Medicine* 126 (1997): 652–53.

72. W. D. Weaver, H. D. White, R. G. Wilcox, et al., "Comparisons of Characteristics and Outcomes Among Women and Men with Acute Myocardial Infarction Treated with Thrombolysis," *Journal of the American Medical Association* 275 (1996): 777–82.

73. National Heart, Lung and Blood Institute, "Women's Health Issues," 14; B. M. Scirica, D. J. Moliterno, N. R. Every, et al., "Differences Between Men and Women in the Management of Unstable Angina Pectoris," *American Journal of Cardiology* 84, no. 10 (1999): 1145–50; Daniel B. Mark, "Sex Bias in Cardiovascular Care: Should Women Be Treated More Like Men?" *Journal of the American Medical*

Association 283, no. 5 (2000): 659–61; M. L. Pearson, K. L. Kahn, E. R. Harrison, et al., "Differences in Quality of Care for Hospitalized Elderly Men and Women," *Journal of the American Medical Association* 268 (1992): 1883–89; N. A. Bickell, K. S. Pieper, K. L. Lee, et al., "Referral Patterns for Coronary Artery Disease Treatment: Gender Bias or Good Clinical Judgment?" *Annals of Internal Medicine* 116 (1999): 791–97; C. Maynard, J. R. Beshansky, J. L. Griffith, and H. P. Selker, "Influence of Sex on the Use of Cardiac Procedures in Patients Presenting to the Emergency Department: A Prospective Multicenter Trial," *Circulation* 94, supp. 9 (1996): 1193–98.

74. D. B. Mark, L. K. Shaw, E. R. DeLong, et al., "Absence of Sex Bias in the Referral of Patients for Cardiac Catheterization," *New England Journal of Medicine* 330 (1994): 1101–6.

75. Delores Kong, "Doubts Heard over Sexual Dysfunction Gathering," *Boston Globe,* October 22, 1999.

76. Hysterectomy Educational Resources and Services Foundation (Bala Cynwyd, PA), http://ccon.com/hers.

77. M. P. Lambden, G. Bellamy, L. Ogburn-Russell, et al., "Women's Sense of Well-being Before and After Hysterectomy," *Journal of Obstetrics, Gynecology and Neonatal Nursing* 26 (1997): 540–48; K. J. Carlson, B. A. Miller, and F. J. Fowler Jr., "The Maine Women's Health Study 1: Outcomes of Hysterectomy," *Obstetrics and Gynecology* 83 (1994): 556–65; H. Virtanen, J. Makinen, T. Tenho, et al., "Effects of Abdominal Hysterectomy on Urinary and Sexual Symptoms," *British Journal of Urology* 72 (1993): 868–72.

78. Julia C. Rhodes, Kristen H. Kjerulff, Patricia W. Langenberg, and Gay M. Guzinski, "Hysterectomy and Sexual Functioning," *Journal of the American Medical Association* 282, no. 20 (1999): 1934–41.

79. Ellen Leopold, *A Darker Ribbon: Breast Cancer, Women and Their Doctors in the Twentieth Century* (Boston: Beacon Press, 1999), 62.

80. Jerome Groopman, review of *A Darker Ribbon* by Ellen Leopold, *New York Times Book Review,* January 9, 2000, 17.

81. Leslie Laurence and Beth Weinhouse, *Outrageous Practices: How Gender Bias Threatens Women's Health* (New Brunswick, NJ: Rutgers University Press, 1994), 282.

82. Christina Hoff Sommers, "The Democrats' Secret Woman Weapon," *Washington Post,* January 5, 1997.

83. Society for Women's Health Research, fund-raising letter, June 16, 1997.

84. Robert Pear, "Research Neglects Women's Health, Studies Find," *New York Times,* April 30, 2000.

85. "Government-Funded Studies Deny Women Key Health Data" (editorial), *USA Today,* May 5, 2000.

86. General Accounting Office, *Women's Health: NIH Has Increased Its Efforts to Include Women in Research,* GAO/HEHS-00-96 (Washington, DC: General Accounting Office, 2000), 8.

87. Sally L. Satel, "Science by Quota," *New Republic* (February 27, 1995): 14–16.

88. A number of conditions apply. According to Dr. Lawrence Friedman of the National Heart, Lung and Blood Institute at NIH (personal communication with the author, June 27, 2000), being in a particular trial is not the only way for someone to be on a drug. First, there is usually more than one ongoing trial for a particular agent (or closely related agents). Second, many trials are conducted with drugs that are FDA-approved for other indications. These drugs may be prescribed for reasons other than the FDA approval (so-called off-label prescribing), including the medical condition under study in a particular trial. Third, there may be trials studying a condition for which the drug in question has been approved; these are comparison trials in which several drugs are being compared against each other and placebo.

89. Food and Drug Administration, "Guideline for the Study and Evaluation of Gender Differences in the Clinical Evaluation of Drugs" (notice), *Federal Register,* July 22, 1993, 39410.

90. L. S. Freedman, M. A. Simon, M. A. Foulkes, et al., "Inclusion of Women and Minorities in Clinical Trials and the NIH Revitalization Act of 1993: The Perspective of NIH Clinical Trialists," *Controlled Clinical Trials* 16 (1995): 277–85.

91. Paul Leber, M.D., personal communication with the author, September 5, 1999.

92. Curtis L. Meinert, "Comments on NIH Clinical Trials Valid Analysis Requirement," *Controlled Clinical Trials* 16 (1995): 304–6.

93. Office of Research on Women's Health, National Institutes of Health, "Implementation of the NIH Guidelines on the Inclusion of Women and Minorities as Subjects in Clinical Research: Comprehensive Report; FY1997 Tracking Data" (May 2000), table 4D; see also Julie E. Buring, "Women in Clinical Trials: A Portfolio for Success," *New England Journal of Medicine* 343 (2000): 505–6.

94. Office of Senator Tom Harkin, "Harkin, Snowe, Mikulski and Waxman Criticize NIH for Failure to Fully Analyze Clinical Data on Women's Health" (press release), May 2, 2000.

95. Ibid.

96. "Six Honored by Society for Outstanding Achievement," *Women's Health Research News* [Society for the Advancement of Women's Health Research] (Fall 1996): 1.

97. In 1999, 35.5 percent of the membership of the American College of Healthcare Executives were women. In their mid-forties on average, members are primarily administrators at the vice president and assistant vice president level at large acute-care health facilities; Peter Kimball (director of research, ACHE), personal communication with the author, June 27, 2000. According to the Association of University Programs in Health Administration, roughly one-third of graduating classes at the master's level have been women since 1992.

98. "Magazine Selects Top Women's Health Centers," *CNN Interactive,* http://cnn.com/-HEALTH/women/9905/31/womens.health.centers, May 31, 1999.

99. Centers for Disease Control, "National Hospital Ambulatory Medical Care Survey," advance data 304 (1997): table 1: Emergency Department Visits; C. A. Green and C. R. Pope, "Gender, Psychosocial Factors and the Use of Medical Services: A Longitudinal Analysis," *Social Science and Medicine* 48 (1999): 1363–72; K. D. Bertakis, R. Azari, L. J. Helms, et al., "Gender Differences in the Utilization of Health Care," *Journal of Family Practice* 49 (2000): 147–52.

100. William Douglas Daniel, M.D., personal communication with the author, October 29, 1998; Michelle G. Curtis, M.D. (University of Texas School of Medicine, Houston), personal communication with the author, February 26, 1999.

101. Bickel, "Women in Academic Medicine."

102. Cathy Young, *Ceasefire!: Why Men and Women Must Join Forces to Achieve Full Equality* (New York: Free Press, 1999).

103. Society for the Advancement of Women's Health Research (now the Society for Women's Health Research), brochure, received January 1997.

104. "Research Office Fills Gender Gap, Backers Say," *USA Today,* October 5, 1999.

105. Edward E. Bartlett, Ph.D., personal communication with the author, January 11, 2000.

Chapter 5

1. Edgar O. Horger, Shirley B. Brown, and Charles Molony Condon, "Cocaine in Pregnancy: Confronting the Problem," *Journal of the South Carolina Medical Association* 86, no. 10 (1990): 527–31.

2. "Jailing Pregnant Drug Users: Does It Help or Hurt?" ABC-TV *Nightline,* June 19, 1990. Note that prior to 1990, if a patient tested positive for cocaine, she was arrested. In 1990 the City of Charleston (Medical University of South Carolina, Solicitor's Office and Charleston City Police) changed the policy to give patients a choice of receiving treatment or being arrested and prosecuted;

Joseph C. Good Jr. (MUSC general counsel), personal communication with the author, January 6, 1998. None of the women arrested was prosecuted.

3. Horger, Brown, and Condon, "Cocaine in Pregnancy."

4. Lynn Paltrow, *Punishing Women for Their Behavior During Pregnancy: An Approach That Undermines Women's Health and Children's Interests* (New York: Center for Reproductive Law and Policy, 1996). Paltrow is now with the National Advocates for Pregnant Women, New York City.

5. Catherine Christophillis, interview with the author, January 26, 1999.

6. Shirley Brown, interview with the author, January 28, 1999.

7. Paltrow, *Punishing Women for Their Behavior During Pregnancy,* 9.

8. George De Leon, "Legal Pressure in Treatment Communities," in *Compulsory Treatment of Drug Abuse: Research and Clinical Practice,* edited by Carl G. Leukfeld and Frank M. Tims, National Institute on Drug Abuse Monograph 86 (Washington, DC: U.S. Government Printing Office, 1988), 160–77, 169.

9. *Crystal Ferguson v. City of Charleston,* CA2:93-2624-12, U.S. Dist. SC, Charleston (1997). The plaintiffs also petitioned the U.S. Supreme Court, claiming that the hospital violated their constitutional protection against unreasonable searches when lower courts decided against them. Their appeal was heard on October 4, 2000, and will probably be decided in 2001, according to the *Washington Post;* see Joan Biskupic, "'Crack Babies' and Rights," *Washington Post,* February 29, 2000, and Linda Greenhouse, "Should a Fetus's Well-Being Override a Mother's Rights?" *New York Times,* September 9, 2000.

10. Charles M. Condon, "Clinton's Cocaine Babies: Why Won't the Administration Let Us Save Our Children?" *Policy Review* (Spring 1995): 12–15.

11. Dorothy E. Roberts, "Punishing Drug Addicts Who Have Babies: Women of Color, Equality, and the Right of Privacy," *Harvard Law Review* 104, no. 7 (1991): 1419–82; see also Dorothy E. Roberts, *Killing the Black Body: Race, Reproduction and the Meaning of Liberty* (New York: Pantheon Books, 1997).

12. Chief Reuben Greenberg, interview with the author, January 28, 1999.

13. *Ferguson v. City of Charleston,* judgment entered September 30, 1997, Charleston, SC, 8, 10.

14. Mary Faith Marshall, testimony before U.S. House, International Affairs and Criminal Justice of the Government Reform and Oversight Committee, Subcommittee on National Security, "Expectant Mothers and Substance Abuse: Intervention and Treatment Challenges for State Governments" (hearing), July 23, 1998.

15. Stephen R. Kandall, *Substance and Shadow: Women and Addiction in the United States* (Cambridge, MA: Harvard University Press, 1996), 298.

16. Francine Feinberg, testimony before U.S. House, International Affairs and Criminal Justice of the Government Reform and Oversight Committee, Subcommittee on National Security, "Expectant Mothers and Substance Abuse: Intervention and Treatment Challenges for State Governments" (hearing), July 23, 1998.

17. Lynn Paltrow, interview with Ted Koppel, "Jailing Pregnant Drug Users: Does It Help or Hurt?" ABC-TV *Nightline,* June 19, 1990.

18. Mary Briody Mahowald, *Genes, Women, Equality* (New York: Oxford University Press, 2000), 25, 27.

19. Ibid., 25.

20. www.harmreduction.org/prince.html.

21. "Mother Dog" column, *Harm Reduction Coalition Communication* (Spring 1997): 23.

22. Linda C. Mayes, Richard H. Granger, Marc H. Bornstein, and Barry Zuckerman, "The Problem of Prenatal Cocaine Abuse: A Rush to Judgment," *Journal of the American Medical Association* 267, no. 3 (1992): 406–8.

23. Barry M. Lester, Linda L. LaGasse, and Ronald Seifer, "Cocaine Exposure and Children: The Meaning of Subtle Effects," *Science* 282 (October 23, 1998): 633–34.

24. National Press Club, Robert Wood Johnson Foundation Substance Abuse Policy Research Program, "Substance Abuse by Pregnant Women," August 11, 1998.

25. Mayes, Granger, Bornstein, and Zuckerman, "The Problem of Prenatal Cocaine Abuse."

26. I. J. Chasnoff, D. R. Griffith, S. MacGregor, et al., "Temporal Patterns of Cocaine Use in Pregnancy: Perinatal Outcomes," *Journal of the American Medical Association* 261, no. 12 (1989): 1741–44.

27. G. Emmet, "What Happened to the 'Crack Babies'?" *Drug Policy Analysis Bulletin,* no. 4 (Washington, DC: Federation of American Scientists, 1998); T. Hawley et al., "Children of Addicted Mothers: Effects of the Crack Epidemic on the Caregiving Environment and the Development of Pre-schoolers," *American Journal of Orthopsychiatry* 65, no. 3 (1995): 364–79.

28. Rita Rubin, "Study: Hands Off Pregnant Drug Users," *USA Today,* August 12, 1998.

29. Joseph A. Califano et al., *Substance Abuse and the American Woman* (New York: National Center on Addiction and Substance Abuse, Columbia University, June 1996), 19.

30. National Committee to Prevent Child Abuse, "The Relationship Between Parental Alcohol or Other Drug Problems and Child Maltreatment," factsheet 14, September 1996.

31. Califano et al., *Substance Abuse and the American Woman,* 16.

32. See Douglas Besharov, "Children of Crack: A Status Report," *Public Welfare* (Winter 1996): 33–37.

33. Califano et al., *Substance Abuse and the American Woman,* 15.

34. National Press Club, Robert Wood Johnson Foundation Substance Abuse Policy Research Program, "Substance Abuse by Pregnant Women," August 11, 1998.

35. Judy Howard, "Barriers to Successful Intervention," in *When Drug Addicts Have Children: Reorienting Child Welfare's Response,* edited by D. Besharov (Washington, DC: Child Welfare League of America/American Enterprise Institute, 1994), 91–100, 98.

36. Mary Utne O'Brien and Sara Segal Loevy, "Barriers to Treatment for Drug Addiction Experienced by Pregnant Women: A Report to the General Accounting Office," task order 90-06, Abt Associates, Chicago Branch, November 1990, 17.

37. Douglas Besharov, "Children of Crack: A Status Report," *Public Welfare* (Winter 1996): 33–37, 34.

38. Besharov, *When Drug Addicts Have Children.*

39. National Center on Addiction and Substance Abuse, Columbia University, "No Safe Haven: Children of Substance Abusing Parents," January 1999, iv.

40. Reuters, "Bid to Sterilize Drug Addicts Is Opposed by California Activists," *Washington Post,* October 21, 1999.

41. Pam Belluck, "Cash-for-Sterilization Plan Draws Addicts and Critics," *New York Times,* July 24, 1999.

42. Barbara Harris, personal communication with the author, December 17, 1997; Anne-Marie O'Neill and Kelly Carter, "Desperate Measures," *People* (September 27, 1999): 145–49.

43. D. B. Marlowe, K. C. Kirby, L. M. Bonieskie, et al., "Assessment of Coercive and Noncoercive Pressures to Enter Drug Abuse Treatment," *Journal of Drug and Alcohol Dependence* 42 (1996): 77–84.

44. O'Brien and Loevy, "Barriers to Treatment for Drug Addiction Experienced by Pregnant Women," 19.

45. Bob Herbert, "Pregnancy and Addiction," *New York Times,* June 11, 1998.

46. Catherine Christophillis, testimony before U.S. House, International Affairs and Criminal Justice of the Government Reform and Oversight Committee, Subcommittee on National Security, "Expectant Mothers and Substance Abuse: Intervention and Treatment Challenges for State Governments" (hearing), July 23, 1998.

47. Dwayne D. Simpson and Susan J. Curry, eds., "Special Issue: Drug Abuse Treatment Outcome Study," *Psychology of Addictive Behaviors* 11, no. 4 (1997): 211–337.

48. E. R. Rahdert, ed., *Treatment for Drug-Exposed Women and Their Children* (Rockville, MD: National Institute on Drug Abuse, 1996), 117. See articles in this volume by J. Howard and L. Beckwith, and by R. Lewis et al.

49. Barbara W. Lex, "Women Civilly Committed to Substance Abuse Treatments in Massachusetts," paper presented at the 29th annual meeting of the American Society for Addiction Medicine, New Orleans, April 16–19, 1998.

50. M. L. Poland, M. P. Dombrowski, J. W. Ager, and R. J. Sokol, "Punishing Pregnant Drug Users: Enhancing the Flight from Treatment," *Drug and Alcohol Depenaence* 31 (1993): 199–203; "Amicus Curiae Brief: *Cornelia Whitner v. South Carolina*," *Hastings Women Law Journal* 9, no. 2 (Summer 1998): 139–60.

51. Data from the Division of Biostatistics, Office of Public Health Statistics and Information Systems, South Carolina Department of Health and Environmental Control, tables 17, 22, 24, 25, 27 series; received April 27, 1999.

52. Horger, Brown, and Condon, "Cocaine in Pregnancy."

53. Centers for Disease Control, "Guidelines for National Human Immunodeficiency Virus Case Surveillance, Including Monitoring for Human Immunodeficiency Virus Infection and Acquired Immunodeficiency Syndrome," *Morbidity and Mortality Weekly Review* 48, RR13 (December 10, 1999): 1–28.

54. Centers for Disease Control, "HIV Testing Among Populations at Risk for HIV Infection—Nine States, November 1995 to December 1996," *Morbidity and Mortality Weekly Review* 47, no. 50 (December 25, 1998): 1086–91.

55. General Accounting Office, "Drug Exposed Infants: A Generation at Risk," GAO/HRD-90-138, June 1990.

56. William J. Domina, testimony before U.S. House, International Affairs and Criminal Justice of the Government Reform and Oversight Committee, Subcommittee on National Security, "Expectant Mothers and Substance Abuse: Intervention and Treatment Challenges for State Governments" (hearing), July 23, 1998.

57. Trish Locklair, R.N., personal communication with the author, January 26, 1999.

58. Barry Zuckerman, Deborah A. Frank, R. Hingson, et al., "Effects of Maternal Marijuana and Cocaine Use on Fetal Growth," *New England Journal of Medicine* 320 (1989): 762–68.

59. Leigh V. Beasley, M.D., personal communication with the author, January 25, 1999.

60. Jo Ann Musto Brink, personal communication with the author, January 25, 1999.

61. Brenda Cummings, personal communication with the author, January 25, 1999.

62. Kiva Greer, personal communication with the author, January 25, 1999.

63. Paula Keller, personal communication with the author, January 25, 1999.

64. Leigh V. Beasley, M.D., personal communication with the author, January 25, 1999.

65. Catherine Christophillis, personal communication with the author, November 14, 1999.

66. Shawn Zeller, "Fetal Abuse Laws Gain Favor," *National Journal* 30, no. 30 (July 25, 1998): 1758.

Chapter 6

1. Pius K. Kamau, "A Case of Mutual Distrust," *Journal of the American Medical Association* 282, no. 5 (1999): 410.

2. Kenneth DeVille, "Defending Diversity: Affirmative Action in Medical Education," *American Journal of Public Health* 89, no. 8 (1999): 1256–61.

3. Deborah Shelton, "A Study in Black and White," *American Medical News* (May 1, 2000): 22.

4. Curtis L. Taylor, "Mistakes in the Past, Fears in the Present: Wary of System, Many Blacks Reluctant to Seek Timely Care," *Newsday,* December 4, 1998. In an article in *PR Newswire* ("Bridging the Gap in Health and Health Care by 2010: What Will It Take?" September 14, 2000), Donna Christian-Christensen, Chair of the Congressional Black Caucus Health Braintrust, says, "It is the decade of racism as expressed in health care."

5. President Bill Clinton, radio address, February 21, 1998.

6. S. A. Optenberg, I. M. Thompson, P. Friedrichs, et al., "Race, Treatment and Long-term Survival from Prostate Cancer in an Equal-Access Medical Care Delivery System," *Journal of the American Medical Association* 274 (1995): 1599–1605; J. A. Dominitz, G. P. Samsa, P. Landsman, and D. Provenzale, "Race, Treatment and Survival Among Colorectal Carcinoma Patients in an Equal-Access Medical

System," *Cancer* 82 (1998): 2312–20; W. J. Mayer and W. P. McWhorter, "Black/White Differences in Nontreatment of Bladder Cancer Patients and Implications for Survival," *American Journal of Public Health* 79 (1989): 772–75.

7. Clinton, radio address, February 21, 1998.

8. Paul Starr, *The Social Transformation of American Medicine* (New York: Basic Books, 1982).

9. R. M. Raup and E. A. Williams, "Negro Students in Medical Schools in the United States," *Journal of Medical Education* 39 (1964): 444–56.

10. Vanessa Northington Gamble, "A Legacy of Distrust: African-Americans and Medical Research," *American Journal of Preventive Medicine* 9, supp. (1993): 35–37.

11. U.S. Commission on Civil Rights, *The Health Care Challenge: Acknowledging Disparity, Confronting Discrimination and Ensuring Equality*, vol. 2, *The Role of Federal Civil Rights Enforcement Efforts* (September 1999), 14.

12. Tatsha Robertson, "Getting to the Heart of Minorities' Health Care," *Boston Globe*, February 28, 1999.

13. Leslie Pickering Francis, "Affirmative Action and the Allocation of Health Care," *Mount Sinai Journal of Medicine* 66, no. 4 (1999): 241–46. Note that the entire quotation reads: "Racism remains the presumptive cause of, and affirmative action the appropriate remedy for, the health care problems minorities face."

14. J. L. Escarce, K. R. Epstein, D. C. Colby, and J. S. Schwartz, "Racial Difference in the Elderly's Use of Medical Procedures and Diagnostic Tests," *American Journal of Public Health* 83 (1993): 948–54; E. A. Mort, J. S. Weissman, and A. M. Epstein, "Physician Discretion and Racial Variation in the Use of Surgical Procedures," *Archives of Internal Medicine* 154 (1994): 761–67; J. Z. Ayanian, I. S. Udvarhelyi, C. A. Gatsonis, et al., "Racial Differences in the Use of Revascularization Procedures After Coronary Angiography," *Journal of the American Medical Association* 269 (1993): 2642–46; Risa B. Burns, Ellen P. Mc-Carthy, Karen M. Freund, et al., "Black Women Receive Less Mammography Even with Similar Use of Primary Care," *Annals of Internal Medicine* 125 (1996): 173–82; Jeff Whittle, Joseph Conigliaro, C. B. Good, and Monica Joswiak, "Do Patient Preferences Contribute to Racial Differences in Cardiovascular Procedure Use?" *Journal of General Internal Medicine* 12 (1997): 267–73; M. E. Gornick, P. W. Eggers, T. W. Reilly, et al., "Effects of Race and Income on Mortality and Use of Services Among Medicare Beneficiaries," *New England Journal of Medicine* 335, no. 11 (1996): 791–99; R. D. Moore, D. Stanton, R. Gopalan, and R. E. Chaisson, "Racial Differences in the Use of Drug Therapy for HIV Disease in an Urban Community," *New England Journal of Medicine* 330 (1994): 763–78. A particularly elegant study by Gail Daumit and her colleagues at Johns Hopkins found that the gap between better-insured white patients and poorly covered black patients disappeared after the black patients reached age sixty-five and began receiving health insurance through Medicare; Gail L. Daumit, Judith A. Hermann, Josef Coresh, and Neil R. Powe, "Use of Cardiovascular Procedures Among Black Persons and White Persons: A Seven-Year Nationwide Study in Patients with Renal Disease," *Annals of Internal Medicine* 130 (1999): 173–82; M. E. Charlson and J. P. Allegrante, "Disparities in the Use of Total Joint Arthroplasty," *New England Journal of Medicine* 342 (2000): 1044–45. Note that in 1990 the AMA Council on Ethical and Judicial Affairs issued opinion 9.121, "Racial Disparities in Health Care."

15. P. B. Bach, L. D. Cramer, J. L. Warren, and C. B. Begg, "Racial Differences in the Treatment of Early-Stage Lung Cancer," *New England Journal of Medicine* 341, no. 16 (1999): 1198–1205.

16. D. E. Campbell and E. R. Greenberg, letter to the editor, *New England Journal of Medicine* 342, no. 7 (2000): 517.

17. Denise Grady, "Racial Discrepancy Is Reported in Surgery for Lung Cancer," *New York Times*, October 14, 1999.

18. K. H. Todd, C. Deaton, A. P. D'Adamo, and L. Goe, "Ethnicity and Analgesic Practice," *Annals of Emergency Medicine* 35 (2000): 11–16.

19. Gabrielle Glaser, "In Treating Patients for Pain, a Racial Gap," *New York Times*, December 28, 1999.

20. John Landsverk, "Patient Race and Ethnicity in Primary Care Management of Child Behavior Problems: An Important Nonfinding," *Medical Care* 37, no. 11 (1999): 1089–91.

21. Kelly J. Kelleher, Cathy D. Moore, George E. Childs, et al., "Patient Race and Ethnicity in Primary Care Management of Child Behavior Problems: A Report from PROS and ASPN," *Medical Care* 37, no. 11 (1999): 1092–1104.

22. K. A. Schulman, J. A. Berlin, W. Harless, et al., "The Effect of Race and Sex on Physicians' Recommendations for Cardiac Catheterization," *New England Journal of Medicine* 340, no. 8 (1999): 618–26; E. D. Peterson, L. K. Shaw, E. R. DeLong, et al., "Racial Variation in the Use of Coronary Revascularization Procedures: Are the Differences Real? Do They Matter?" *New England Journal of Medicine* 336 (1997): 480–86; M. Laouri, R. L. Kravitz, W. J. French, et al., "Underuse of Cardiac Procedures: Application of a Clinical Method," *Journal of the American College of Cardiologists* 29 (1997): 891–97.

23. "America in Black and White: Health Care, the Great Divide," ABC-TV *Nightline*, February 24, 1999.

24. Schulman, Berlin, Harless, et al., "The Effect of Race and Sex on Physicians' Recommendations," 624.

25. "Medical Treatment Based on Color of the Skin: Study Shows Doctors Have Unconscious Bias," ABC-TV *World News This Morning*, February 25, 1999.

26. Peter Jennings, ABC-TV *World News Tonight*, February 24, 1999, as reported in "Minority Health: Study Confirms Heart Test 'Bias,'" *American Health Line* (February 25, 1999).

27. "America in Black and White: Health Care, the Great Divide," ABC-TV *Nightline*, February 24, 1999.

28. "Cardiac Testing: Study Finds Women, Blacks Are Being Shortchanged," *Chicago Tribune*, March 18, 1999.

29. "Health Care: It's Better If You're White," *The Economist* (February 27, 1999): 28–29.

30. "Institutionalized Racism in Health Care" (editorial), *Lancet* 353, no. 9155 (1999): 765.

31. Lucian L. Leape, Lee H. Hilborne, Robert Bell, et al., "Underuse of Cardiac Procedures: Do Women, Ethnic Minorities and the Uninsured Fail to Receive Needed Revascularization?" *Annals of Internal Medicine* 130 (1999): 183–92.

32. Lisa M. Schwartz, Steven Woloshin, and M. Gilbert Welch, "Misunderstandings About the Effects of Race and Sex on Physicians' Referrals for Cardiac Catheterization," *New England Journal of Medicine* 341, no. 4 (1999): 279–83. According to a letter to the editor (ibid., 286), K. A. Schulman, J. A. Berlin, and J. J. Escarce report that the average referrals per actor-patients were: white fifty-five-year-old male referred by 91.1 percent of doctors; white seventy-year-old male referred by 90 percent; black fifty-five-year-old male referred by 91.1 percent; black seventy-year-old male referred by 90 percent; white fifty-five-year-old female referred by 92.2 percent; white seventy-year-old female referred by 88.9 percent; black fifty-year-old female referred by 84.4 percent; and black seventy-year-old female referred by 73.3 percent. It is the seventy-year-old black female actor-patient in particular who garnered the noticeably lower rate of referrals. It is not clear why this was so. Because there was only one actor-patient per category, it is possible that this particular woman was not very convincing in her portrayal of a cardiac patient.

33. According to Schwartz et al., "The authors [Schulman and his colleagues] chose to summarize the relative chance of referral for blacks as compared with whites using an odds ratio—literally, the ratio of the odds in favor of being referred for catheterization for blacks to the odds for whites. [That would mean that] the odds that blacks would be referred for catheterization were 40 percent lower than the odds of referral for whites. The use of the odds ratio is unfortunate. Few people think in terms of odds or encounter them in daily life. Perhaps for this reason, many people tend to equate odds with probability (the most familiar way to characterize chance) and thus to equate odds ratios with risk ratios. . . . Because the study by Schulman et al. involved a very common event (84.7 [85 rounded] percent of blacks and 90.6 [91 rounded] percent of whites were referred for cardiac

catheterization), the overstatement in this case was extreme. The reported odds ratio of .6 actually corresponds to a risk ratio of .93 [85 percent divided by 91 percent]. Inappropriately equating odds ratios with risk ratios led to the mistaken impression that blacks had a 40 percent lower probability of referral than whites, whereas in fact, the probability of referral for blacks was 7 percent lower [1.0 minus .93]. In this case, the failure to distinguish between odds ratios and risk ratios had profound consequences for how the magnitude of the difference in referral rates for blacks and whites was portrayed"; ibid., 280.

34. Ibid.

35. Gregory D. Curfman and Jerome P. Kassirer, editors' note, *New England Journal of Medicine* 341, no. 4 (1999): 287. "We should not have allowed the use of odds ratios in the Abstract," wrote Curfman and Kassirer. See also Frank Davidoff (ibid., 286), who wrote, "It is unfortunate that the authors did not emphasize the simpler, more direct measure," referring to relative risk.

36. Kevin A. Schulman, J. A. Berlin, and J. J. Escarce, authors' reply, *New England Journal of Medicine* 341, no. 4 (1999): 286.

37. Kevin A. Schulman, M.D., personal communication with the author, August 9, 1999.

38. Kathleen Fackelmann, "Does Unequal Treatment Really Have Roots in Racism?" *USA Today,* September 16, 1999.

39. John Leo, "Shocking, but Not True," *U.S. News & World Report,* November 22, 1999; Jennifer Greenstein, "The Heart of the Matter," *Brill's Content* (October 1999): 40.

40. "Key Facts: Race, Ethnicity and Medical Care," *Henry J. Kaiser Family Foundation* (October 1999): 30.

41. Edward Guadagnoli, John Z. Ayanian, Gary Gibbons, et al., "The Influence of Race on the Use of Surgical Procedures for Treatment of Peripheral Vascular Disease of the Lower Extremities," *Archives of General Surgery* 130 (1995): 381–86.

42. B. J. McNeil, R. Weichselbaum, and S. G. Pauker, "Fallacy of the Five-Year Survival in Lung Cancer," *New England Journal of Medicine* 299 (1978): 1397–1401; Eugene Z. Oddone, Ronnie D. Horner, Tiffiny Diers, et al., "Understanding Racial Variation in the Use of Carotid Endarterectomy: The Role of Aversion to Surgery," *Journal of the National Medical Association* 90 (1998): 25–33; A. D. Schecter, P. J. Goldschmidt-Clermont, G. McKee, et al., "Influence of Gender, Race and Education on Patient Preferences and Receipt of Cardiac Catheterization Among Coronary Care Unit Patients," *American Journal of Cardiology* 78 (1996): 996–1001.

43. Ronnie D. Horner, Eugene Z. Oddone, and David B. Matchar, "Theories Explaining Racial Differences in the Utilization of Diagnostic and Therapeutic Procedures for Cerebrovascular Disease," *Milbank Quarterly* 73, no. 3 (1995): 443–62.

44. Deborah Shelton, "A Study in Black and White," *American Medical News,* May 1, 2000, 23.

45. W. W. O'Neill, "Multivessel Balloon Angioplasty Should Be Abandoned in Diabetic Patients," *Journal of the American College of Cardiology* 31 (1998): 20–22; S. G. Ellis and C. R. Narins, "Problem of Angioplasty in Diabetics," *Circulation* 96 (1997): 1707–10.

46. Leape, Hilborne, Bell, et al., "Underuse of Cardiac Procedures." Leape and his colleagues defined need using the RAND Appropriateness Method, which they describe in detail in the article's appendix.

47. Otis Brawley and Kevin A. Knopf, "Cancer in Special Populations," forthcoming in *Journal of the National Cancer Institute.*

48. L. A. Maiman and M. H. Becker, "The Health Belief Model: Origins and Correlates in Psychological Theory," *Health Education Monographs* 2 (1974): 336–53.

49. Clive O. Callender, M.D., personal communication with the author, August 9, 1999; see also Callender's testimony before the House Commerce Committee, Subcommittee on Health and the Environment, and the Senate Labor and Human Resources Committee, June 18, 1998.

50. R. Ozminkowski, A. J. White, A. Hassol, and M. Murphy, "Minimizing Racial Disparity Regarding Receipt of a Cadaver Kidney Transplant," *American Journal of Kidney Diseases* 30 (1997):

749–59; *Organ Procurement and Transplantation: Assessing Current Policies and Potential Impact of the DHHS Final Rule* (Washington, DC: National Academy Press, 1999), 38; P. J. Held, M. V. Pauly, R. R. Bovbjerg, et al., "Access to Kidney Transplantation: Has the United States Eliminated Income and Racial Differences?" *Archives of Internal Medicine* 148 (1988): 2594–2600; "Black Ministers Urging Congregation to Become Organ, Tissue and Blood Donors," *Transplant News* (August 31, 1998); Holly G. Franz, Jessica Drachman, William DeJong, et al., "Public Attitudes Toward Organ Donation: Implications for OPO Coordinators," *Journal of Transplant Coordination* 5 (1995): 50–54.

51. Wayne B. Arnason, "Directed Donation: The Relevance of Race," *Hastings Center Report* (November-December 1991): 13–19; Held, Pauly, Bovbjerg, et al., "Access to Kidney Transplantation"; P. McNamara, E. Guadagnoli, M. J. Evanisko, et al., "Correlates of Support for Organ Donation Among Three Ethnic Groups," *Clinical Transplantation* 13 (1999): 45–50. Although the organ allocation system does not earmark donations by race, it does ensure histocompatibility, which tends to favor same-race donor-recipient pairs. The system also allows cross donations whenever an acceptable match can be found; as a result, black patients often receive kidneys from white donors because whites are the source of most donated kidneys.

52. Arnason, "Directed Donation."

53. David Barton Smith, *Health Care Divided: Race and Healing a Nation* (Ann Arbor: University of Michigan Press, 1999), 27.

54. Jim Warren, "Transplant Community Outraged: Farrakhan Says That Whites Condone Black-on-Black Killings Because It's a Source of Transplantable Organs," *Transplant News* (May 13, 1994); Ian Ayers, Laura G. Dooley, and Robert S. Gaston, "Unequal Racial Access to Kidney Transplantation," *Vanderbilt Law Review* 46 (May 1993): 805–63.

55. U.S. Commission on Civil Rights, *The Role of Federal Civil Rights Enforcement Efforts,* 111.

56. William F. Owen Jr., Glenn M. Chertow, J. Michael Lazarus, and Edmund G. Lowrie, "Dose of Hemodialysis and Survival: Differences by Race and Sex," *Journal of the American Medical Association* 280 (1998): 1764–68. For the death rate on those on waiting lists, see htpp://www.unos.org/-Data/anrpt98/ar98_table66_02-ki.htm.

57. United Network for Organ Sharing, "1999 Organ Procurement and Transplantation Network Annual Report," http://www.unos.org/Data/anrpt99/ar99_table28_03_kid.htm.

58. Ozminkowski et al., "Minimizing Racial Disparity Regarding Receipt of a Cadaver Kidney Transplant."

59. In data provided by the U.S. Scientific Registry and Organ Procurement and Transplantation Network (SR&OPTN) (1999), table 52 shows individuals on a waiting list in 1998 (20,616 whites; 14,923 blacks); table 26 shows living kidney donor recipients (2,953 whites; 542 blacks); and table 25 shows cadaveric kidney recipients (4,462 whites, 2,152 blacks). Thus, 7,415 whites received kidneys out of 20,616—or 36 percent of waiting-list whites—compared to 2,694 blacks who received kidneys out of 14,932—or 18 percent of waiting-list blacks; see www.unos.org/frame_Default.asp?Category=Search.

60. Poor patients who become ill with end-stage renal disease can get Medicaid, which covers the cost of post-transplantation medications indefinitely, whereas Medicare payment stops after three years.

61. United Network for Organ Sharing (Richmond, VA), "Background: Problems and Concerns in Equitable Organ Allocation: Statement of Principles and Objectives—Appendix D," http://204.127.237.11/eg_bkgnd.htm.

62. Fred P. Sanfilippo, William K. Vaughn, Thomas G. Peters, et al., "Factors Affecting the Waiting Time of Cadaveric Kidney Transplant Candidates in the U.S.," *Journal of the American Medical Association* 267 (1992): 247–52; G. C. Alexander and A. R. Sehgal, "Barriers to Cadaveric Renal Transplantation Among Blacks, Women and the Poor," *Journal of the American Medical Association* 280 (1998): 1148–52.

63. John Z. Ayanian, Paul D. Cleary, Joel S. Weissman, and Arnold M. Epstein, "The Effect of Patients' Preferences on Racial Differences in Access to Renal Transplantation," *New England Journal*

of Medicine 341 (1999): 1661–69. The researchers found no association between referral and patient's age, treatment facility, health status, concurrent illness, cause of renal failure or place of residence.

64. Edward Guadagnoli, P. McNamara, M. J. Evanisko, et al., "The Influence of Race on Approaching Families for Organ Donation and Their Decision to Donate," *American Journal of Public Health* 89 (1999): 244–27.

65. Franz, Drachman, DeJong, et al., "Public Attitudes Toward Organ Donation."

66. William DeJong, Holley G. Franz, Susan M. Wolfe, et al., "Requesting Organ Donation: An Interview Study of Donor and Non-Donor Families," *American Journal of Critical Care* 7 (1999): 13–23.

67. Ibid.; Steven L. Gortmaker, Carol L. Beasley, Ellen Sheehy, et al., "Improving the Request Process to Increase Family Consent for Organ Donation," *Journal of Transplant Coordination* 8 (1998): 210–17.

68. UNOS Histocompatibility Committee, "The National Kidney Distribution System: Striving for Equitable Use of a Scarce Resource" (UNOS update), August 1995.

69. Joel D. Kallich, John L. Adams, Phoebe Lindsey Barton, and Karen L. Spritzer, *Access to Cadaveric Kidney Transplantation* (Santa Monica, CA: Rand, 1993), xv.

70. According to the nephrologist Robert Gaston of the University of Alabama School of Medicine, "Current data indicate that the benefits of partial matching are becoming more difficult to document. In the absence of a six-antigen match, being mismatched contributes very little to whether or not one's transplant is likely to succeed"; personal communication with the author, June 16, 2000.

71. R. H. Kerman, P. M. Kimball, C. T. Van Buren, et al., "Possible Contribution of Pre-transplant Immune Responder Status to Renal Allograft Survival Difference of Black Versus White Recipients," *Transplantation* 51 (1991): 338–42; S. Hariharan, T. J. Schroeder, and M. R. Frist, "Effect of Race on Renal Transplant Outcome," *Clinical Transplantation* 7 (1993): 235–39; B. L. Kasiske, J. F. Neylan III, R. R. Riggio, et al., "The Effect of Race on Access and Outcome in Transplantation," *New England Journal of Medicine* 342 (1991): 302–7.

72. Glenn M. Chertow and Edgar L. Milford, "Poor Graft Survival in African-American Transplant Recipients Cannot Be Explained by HLA Mismatching," *Advances in Renal Replacement Therapy* 4 (1997): 40–45.

73. Starting in 1995 new immunosuppressants (drugs that help prevent rejection) became available. This breakthrough may not only improve survival after transplantation for black patients but obviate the need for tight antigen matching, and thus move blacks more quickly up the waiting list. Despite the tremendous promise of these drugs, the clinical verdict on their success will not be in for several years, because it takes at least two years after a transplant to be certain that a kidney will function over the long term; Clive O. Callender, M.D., personal communication with the author, August 9, 1999.

74. "U.S. Facts About Transplantation" (critical data), www.unos.org/Newsroom/critdata_main.htm#transplants.

75. United Network for Organ Sharing, 1999 annual report, tables 17, 52, http://www.unos.org/Data/anrpt99/ar99_table52_02_ki.htm.

76. Maritza Rozon-Solomon and Lewis Burrows, "'Tis Better to Receive Than to Give': The Relative Failure of the African-American Community to Provide Organs for Transplantation," *Mount Sinai Journal of Medicine* 66, no. 4 (1999): 273–76; Kasiske, Neylan, Riggio, et al., "The Effect of Race on Access and Outcome in Transplantation." It should be noted that in 1997 whites represented half of all people on the waiting list, donated about three-quarters of the cadaver kidneys and represented 57 percent of the cadaver kidney recipients; UNOS 1999 annual report.

77. United Network for Organ Sharing, "UNOS Critical Data: Number of U.S. Transplants by Organ and Donor Type," http://www.unos.org/Newsroom/critdata_transplants_ustx.htm; UNOS, "1999 SR&OPTN Annual Report: Living Donor Characteristics 1989–98," http://www.unos.org/Data/anrpt99/ar99_table17_02-kld.htm. In 1998 the black living kidney donation rate was 438, about one-sixth the white donation rate of 2,559 (UNOS table 17).

78. UNOS 1999 annual report, tables 11, 25, 52.

79. Rozon-Solomon and Burrows, "'Tis Better to Receive Than to Give,'" 274.

80. American Medical Association, "Enhancing the Cultural Competence of Physicians: AMA Report of the Council on Medical Education," report 5–A–98 (May 30, 1998), www.ama-assn.org/meetings/public/annual98/report/cme/cmerpts.htm.

81. Anne Fadiman, *The Spirit Catches You and You Fall Down: A Hmong Child, Her American Doctors and the Collision of Two Cultures* (New York: Farrar, Straus and Giroux, 1997).

82. Kaiser Permanente, *Asian and Pacific Island American Population: A Provider Handbook* (Menlo Park, CA: Kaiser Permanente, 1996), 15.

83. Ibid.

84. Kaiser Permanente, *Latino Population: A Provider Handbook* (Menlo Park, CA: Kaiser Permanente, 1996), 36.

85. Ibid., 8.

86. Jennifer Bush (AAMC), personal communication with the author, June 30, 2000.

87. U.S. Public Health Service, Office of Minority Health, 1995 statement.

88. Alliance for Health Reform, "Shrinking the Gap: Reducing Disparities in Minority Health Coverage and Care" (conference), Washington, DC, November 17, 1999.

89. Mike Mitka, "The Bridge at Ann Arbor: Japanese Health," *Journal of the American Medical Association* 283, no. 22 (2000): 2921–22.

90. Louis Harris and Associates, *Health Care Services and Minority Groups: A Comparative Survey of Whites, African-Americans, Hispanics and Asian Americans,* study 932028 (New York: Commonwealth Fund, 1994), table 1–7.

91. Ibid., table 1–17.

92. Ibid., table 1–18.

93. Ibid., table 1–7.

94. Ibid., table 4–10.

95. Ibid., table 3–27.

96. Ibid., table 4–10.

97. Ibid., table 4–14.

98. Ibid., table 4–10.

99. Ibid., table 1–3.

100. Frederick Schneiders Research, "Perceptions of How Race and Ethnic Background Affect Medical Care," focus group conducted for the Henry J. Kaiser Family Foundation, October 1999, 4.

101. Henry J. Kaiser Family Foundation, "Race, Ethnicity and Medical Care: A Survey of Public Perceptions and Experiences" (October 1999), 15. Also note that even though 82 percent of African Americans said their health care was excellent or good, 64 percent of them said they thought whites got better care than they did (9).

102. Ibid., 17.

103. Ibid., 22.

104. Erlich Transcultural Consultants, "New America Wellness: Morehouse College of Medicine Multiethnic Healthcare Attitudinal Research," conducted March 1999; available from Stedman Graham and Partners, New York (212–727–5000). This finding correlated closely with the 27 percent of black respondents who did in fact have a black doctor. Only one in ten whites of this nationally representative sample expressed a preference for a white doctor, though the vast majority had one.

105. A. B. Bindman, K. Grumbach, K. Vranizan, et al., "Selection and Exclusion of Primary Care Physicians by Managed Care Organizations," *Journal of the American Medical Association* 279 (1998): 675–79.

106. E. R. Mackenzie, L. S. Taylor, and R. Lavizzo-Mourey, "Experiences of Ethnic Minority Primary Care Physicians with Managed Care: A National Survey," *American Journal of Managed Care* 5 (1999): 1251–64.

107. National Medical Association, press conference, Washington, DC, January 24, 2000.

108. PBS-TV, *NewsHour with Jim Lehrer,* January 25, 2000.

109. Joel C. Cantor, Lois Bergeisen, and Laurence C. Baker, "Effect of Intensive Educational Program for Minority College Students and Recent Graduates on the Probability of Acceptance to Medical School," *Journal of the American Medical Association* 280 (1998): 772–76.

110. Laura Meckler, "Panel: Diversify Medical Workforce," Associated Press, December 9, 1998. This rationale for preferences was also put forth in the famous 1976 reverse discrimination case *Regents of the University of California v. Bakke*; see Stanley Mosk, "For Bakke," in *Racial Preference and Racial Justice: The New Affirmative Action Controversy,* edited by R. Nieli (Washington, DC: Ethics and Public Policy, 1991), 159–66.

111. In 1992 the AAMC introduced an initiative called "Project 3000 by 2000" whose goal was to see three thousand underrepresented minority students enter medical school by the year 2000.

112. Jeffrey Mervis, "Wanted: A Better Way to Boost Numbers of Minority Ph.D.s," *Science* 28 (1998): 1268–70.

113. Randal C. Archibold, "Applications to Medical Schools Decline for Second Straight Year," *New York Times,* September 2, 1999; Holcomb B. Noble, "Struggling to Bolster Minorities in Medicine," *New York Times,* September 29, 1998.

114. M. Komaromy, K. Grumbach, M. Drake, et al., "The Role of Black and Hispanic Physicians in Providing Health Care for Underserved Populations," *New England Journal of Medicine* 334 (1996): 1305–10; G. Xu, S. K. Fields, C. Laine, et al., "The Relationship Between the Race and Ethnicity of Generalist Physicians and Their Care for Underserved Patients," *American Journal of Public Health* 87 (1997): 817–22; E. Moy and B. A. Bartman, "Physician Race and Care of Minority and Medically Indigent Patients," *Journal of the American Medical Association* 273 (1995): 1515–20; Joel Cantor, "Physician Service to the Underserved: Implications for Affirmative Action in Medical Education," *Inquiry* 33 (Summer 1996): 167–80.

115. MC, *Minority Graduates of U.S. Medical Schools: Trends, 1950–1988* (Washington, DC: AAMC, 2000), 5.

116. Barbara Barzansky, Harry S. Jonas, and Sylvia I. Etzel, "Educational Programs in U.S. Medical Schools, 1998–1999," *Journal of the American Medical Association* 282 (1999): 840–46.

117. Robert G. Petersdorf, M.D., "Not a Choice, an Obligation," paper presented at the plenary session of the 102nd meeting of the American Association of Medical Colleges, Washington, DC, November 10, 1991.

118. Donald L. Libby, Zijun Zhou, and David A. Kindig, "Will Minority Physician Supply Meet U.S. Needs?" *Health Affairs* 16 (1997): 205–14.

119. Kevin Grumbach, Elizabeth Mertz, and Janet Coffman, "Underrepresented Minorities in Medical Education in California," California Center for Health Workforce Studies at the University of California, San Francisco (March 1999), report available at http://futurehealth.ucsf.edu. Nationwide, minority applications dropped 13 percent from 1996 to 1998. In large part, though not exclusively, the decrease was due to the California initiative and to race no longer being considered a factor in medical school admission in three states (Texas, Louisiana and Mississippi) in the wake of the 1996 Hopwood case. Even though minority applications again declined from 1998 to 1999, there is no evidence that the pool of potential minority applicants is shrinking. The percentage of black and Hispanic students getting bachelor of science degrees has remained constant, as have those races' percentage of college graduates; Ella Cleveland (AAMC Division of Community and Minority Programs), personal communication with the author, January 6, 2000. No one really understands why medical school is relatively unpopular among these students. Perhaps some are discouraged by the high educational debt they will assume or by the loss of physician autonomy in the world of managed care. Interestingly, not all of these developments were a result of Proposition 209 and Hopwood. First, across the country applications from whites have been going down as well; there was a 6 percent drop in all applicants from 1998 to 1999, the third straight year of decline. Second, the decline in minority appli-

cants in California actually started two years before passage of Proposition 209. Third, at California's three *private* medical schools, which were unaffected by the new law, there was also a large drop in minority applications (25 percent) after its passage.

120. Michael J. Scotti Jr., "Medical School Admission Criteria: The Needs of Patients Matter," *Journal of the American Medical Association* 278 (1997): 1196–97.

121. D. M. Carlisle, J. E. Gardner, and H. Liu, "The Entry of Underrepresented Minority Students into U.S. Medical Schools: An Evaluation of Recent Trends," *American Journal of Public Health* 88 (1998): 1314–18.

122. Randall Morgan, "War on Affirmative Action," *Clinical Psychiatry News* (October 1998): 21.

123. Gary C. Dennis, "President's Year in Review," *Journal of the National Medical Association* 91 (1999): 437–38.

124. H. Jack Geiger, "Ethnic Cleansing in the Groves of Academe," *American Journal of Public Health* 88 (1998): 1299–1300, 1299.

125. M. J. O'Sullivan, P. D. Peterson, G. B. Cox, and J. Kirkeby, "Ethnic Populations: Community Mental Health Services Ten Years Later," *American Journal of Community Psychology* 17 (1989): 17–30; Robert Rosenheck and Catherine L. Seibyl, "Participation and Outcome in a Residential Treatment and Work Therapy Program for Addictive Disorders: The Effects of Race," *American Journal of Psychiatry* 155 (1998): 1029–34; S. Sue, D. C. Fijino, L. Hu, et al., "Community Mental Health Services for Ethnic Minorities Groups: A Test of the Cultural Responsiveness Hypothesis," *American Psychologist* 59 (1991): 553–40; R. A. Rosenheck and A. F. Fontana, "Race and Outcome of Treatment for Veterans Suffering from PTSD," *Journal of Traumatic Stress* 9 (1996): 343–51.

126. Matthew J. Chinman, Julie Lam, and Robert A. Rosenheck, "Clinician–Case Manager Racial Matching in a Program for Homeless Persons with Serious Mental Illness," *Psychiatric Services* 51 (2000): 1265–72.

127. Lisa Cooper-Patrick, Joseph J. Gallo, Junius J. Gonzales, et al., "Race, Gender and Partnership in the Patient-Physician Relationship," *Journal of the American Medical Association* 282 (1999): 583–89. No data were provided to show whether patients' perceptions of being satisfied actually translated into objective measures of improved health, though it is well established that a good rapport with one's doctor is associated with better treatment compliance.

128. Senator Edward M. Kennedy, press release announcing introduction of the Health Care Fairness Act of 1999, November 4, 1999.

129. These differences were statistically different.

130. Sherrie H. Kaplan, Barbara Gandek, Sheldon Greenfield, et al., "Patient and Visit Characteristics Related to Physicians' Participatory Decision-making Style," *Medical Care* 33 (1995): 1176–87.

131. Sherrie H. Kaplan, Sheldon Greenfield, Barbara Gandek, et al., "Characteristics of Physicians with Participatory Decision-making Styles," *Annals of Internal Medicine* 124 (1996): 497–504.

132. Bernard D. Davis, *Storm over Biology: Essays on Science, Sentiment and Public Policy* (Buffalo, NY: Prometheus Books, 1986), 174.

133. Ibid.

134. Thomas R. Dye, *Race as an Admissions Factor in Florida's Public Law and Medical Schools* (Tallahassee: Lincoln Center, 1999).

135. See University of California Admissions, http://www.acusd.edu/~e_cook. Despite these marked race-based advantages in admission, the U.S. Commission on Civil Rights charges that medical schools discriminate against minority applicants. Its 1999 report to Congress and the White House bemoans "the persistent yet baffling denial of the social, economic, and historical realities depriving our medical profession of minority physicians"; U.S. Commission on Civil Rights, *The Role of Federal Civil Rights Enforcement Efforts*, 116.

136. Ward Connerly, "My Fight Against Race Preferences: A Quest Toward 'Creating Equal,'" *Chronicle of Higher Education* (March 10, 2000): B6.

137. Cited in Institute of Medicine, *Balancing the Scales of Opportunity: Ensuring Racial and Ethnic Diversity in the Health Professions* (Washington, DC: National Academy Press, 1994), 24.

138. Henry W. Foster Jr., "Reaching Parity for Minority Medical Students: A Possibility or a Pipe Dream?" *Journal of the National Medical Association* 88 (1996): 17–21.

139. American Association of Medical Colleges, *Minority Students in Medical Education: Facts and Figures* IX (Washington, DC: AAMC, 1998).

140. Beth Dawson, Carolyn Iwamoto, Linette Postell Ross, et al., "Performance on the National Board of Medical Examiners Part 1 Examination by Men and Women of Different Race and Ethnicity," *Journal of the American Medical Association* 272 (1994): 674–79.

141. G. Xu, S. K. Fields, C. Laine, et al., "The Relationship Between Race/Ethnicity of Generalist Physicians and Their Care for Underserved Populations," *American Journal of Public Health* 87 (1997): 817–22.

142. Rebecca S. Miller, Marvin R. Dunn, and Thomas Richter, "Graduate Medical Education, 1998–1999: A Closer Look," *Journal of the American Medical Association* 282 (1999): 855–60. According to a 2000 study by the AAMC, belonging to an underrepresented minority is a risk factor for becoming a "problem resident." David C. Yao and Scott M. Wright, "National Survey of Internal Medicine Residency Program Directors Regarding Problem Residents," *Journal of the American Medical Association* 284, no. 9 (2000): 1099–1104.

143. Dawson, Iwamoto, Ross, et al., "Performance on the National Board of Medical Examiners."

144. S. N. Keith, R. M. Bell, and A. P. Williams, "Assessing the Outcome of Affirmative Action in Medical School: A Study of the Class of 1975," Rand Corporation publication R–3481–CWF, August 1987.

145. Robyn Tamblyn, Michael Abrahamowicz, Carlos Brailovsky, et al., "Association Between Licensing Examination Scores and Resource Use and Quality of Care in Primary Care Practice," *Journal of the American Medical Association* 280 (1998): 989–96.

146. P. G. Ramsey, J. D. Carline, T. S. Inui, et al., "Predictive Validity of Certification by the American Board of Internal Medicine," *Annals of Internal Medicine* 110 (1989): 719–26.

147. Vera Taylor and George S. Rust, "The Needs of Students from Diverse Cultures," *Academic Medicine* 74 (1999): 302–3.

148. Institute of Medicine, *Balancing the Scales of Opportunity*, 2.

149. American Medical Student Association, "Minority Medical Education: Assessment Tool and Guidebook," http://www.amsa.org/programs/mededtool.htm.

150. Association of American Medical Colleges, "Expanded Minority Admission Exercise," http://www.aamc.org/meded/minority/emae/start.htm.

151. On the MCATs' predictive validity, see S.M. Case et al., "Performance of the Class of 1994 in the New Era of USMLE," *Academic Medicine* 71, no. 10 (1996): S91–93; K. L. Huff, J. A. Koenig, M. M. Treptau, and S. G. Sireci, "Validity of MCAT Scores for Predicting Clerkship Performance of Medical Students Grouped by Race and Sex," *Academic Medicine* 74, no. 10 (1999): S41–44; K. L. Huff and D. Fang, "When Are Students at Most Risk in Encountering Academic Difficulty? A Study of the 1992 Matriculants to U.S. Medical Schools," *Academic Medicine* 74, no. 4 (1999): 454–60; J. A. Koenig, S. G. Sireci, and A. Wiley, "Evaluating the Predictive Validity of MCAT Scores Across Diverse Applicant Groups," *Academic Medicine* 73, no. 10 (1998): 1095–1106; A. Tekian et al., "Baseline Longitudinal Data of Undergraduate Medical Students at Risk," *Academic Medicine* 73, no. 10 (1998): S38–40. On the relationship between noncognitive variables and medical school performance, see C. L. Elam et al., "Challenging the System: Admission Issues for At-Risk Students, Admissions Committees," *Academic Medicine* 74, no. 10 (1999): S58–61; C. T. Webb et al., "The Impact of Non-Academic Variables on Performance at Two Medical Schools," *Journal of the National Medical Association* 89, no. 3 (1997): 173–80; W. E. Selacek and D. O. Prieto, "Predicting Minority Students' Success in Medical School," *Academic Medicine* 65, no. 3 (1990): 161–65; B. Mavis and K. Doig, "The Value of Non-Cognitive Fac-

tors in Predicting Students' First-Year Academic Probation," *Academic Medicine* 73, no. 2 (1998): 201–3; H. Shen and A. L. Comrey, "Predicting Medical Students' Academic Performances by Their Cognitive Abilities and Personality Characterictics," *Academic Medicine* 72, no. 9 (1997): 781–86.

152. Robert C. Davidson and Ernest L. Lewis, "Affirmative Action and Other Special Consideration Admissions at the University of California, Davis, School of Medicine," *Journal of the American Medical Association* 278 (1997): 1153–58.

153. Foster, "Reaching Parity for Minority Medical Students," 20.

154. Human Resources and Services Administration, *Minorities in Medicine: Council on Graduate Medical Education Twelfth Report* (Washington, DC: U.S. Department of Health and Human Services, May 1998).

155. AAMC, *Minority Graduates of U.S. Medical Schools,* 25. Since 1970 Asian students increased their representation among medical school graduates by 46-fold, African Americans by 7-fold and Hispanics by 11-fold. In terms of absolute numbers, there were 63 Asians in the 1970 graduating class of 8,367; by 1998 there were 2,849 out of 15,949. In 1970 there were 188 graduating African Americans, and in 1998 there were 1,211. In 1970 there were 86 graduating Hispanic students, and in 1998 there were 1,024.

156. E. L. Hannan, "The Relationship Between Volume and Outcome on Health Care," *New England Journal of Medicine* 340 (1999): 1677–79; E. B. Keeler, L. V. Rubinstein, K. L. Kahn, et al., "Hospital Characteristics and Quality of Care," *Journal of the American Medical Association* 268 (1992): 1709–14; E. B. Edwards, J. P. Roberts, M. A. McBride, et al., "The Effect of the Volume of Procedures at Transplantation Centers on Mortality After Liver Transplantation," *New England Journal of Medicine* 341 (1999): 2049–53.

157. K. L. Kahn, M. L. Pearson, E. R. Harrison, K. A. Desmond, et al., "Health Care for Black and Poor Hospitalized Medicare Patients," *Journal of the American Medical Association* 271 (1994): 1169–74.

158. Leonard D. Baer, Thomas C. Ricketts, and Thomas R. Konrad, "International Medical Graduates in Rural, Underserved Areas," *Findings Brief, Cecil G. Sheps Center for Health Services Research* [University of North Carolina at Chapel Hill] (May 1998): 1–4.

159. Jay Greene, "Primary Push," *American Medical News* (March 13, 2000): 10–12.

160. T. P. Weil, "Attracting Qualified Physicians to Underserved Areas," *Physician Executive* 25 (1999): 53–63.

Chapter 7

1. Melodie J. Peet, opening remarks at the Maine Trauma Advisory Groups Statewide Invitational Forum, Augusta, November 18, 1996.

2. Ann Jennings (Department of Mental Health, Mental Retardation and Substance Abuse Services, Office of Trauma Services), "Comprehensive Strategic Action Plan for Creating a System of Care Responsive to the Needs of Trauma Survivors" (April 1998), 3.

3. National Association of State Mental Health Program Directors, "Position Statement on Services and Supports to Trauma Survivors" (December 1998).

4. Ellen Bass and Laura Davis, *The Courage to Heal: A Guide for Women Survivors of Child Sexual Abuse* (New York: HarperCollins, 1992), 22.

5. Judith Lewis Herman, *Trauma and Recovery: The Aftermath of Violence—From Domestic Abuse to Political Terror* (New York: Basic Books, 1992), 1.

6. Ibid., 9.

7. Sandra Bloom, *Creating Sanctuary: Toward an Evolution of Sane Societies* (New York: Routledge, 1997), 119.

8. David Finklehor, "Improving Research, Policy and Practice to Understand Child Sexual Abuse," *Journal of the American Medical Association* 280, no. 21 (December 2, 1998): 1864–65; Jeffrey G. John-

son, Patricia Cohen, Jocelyn Brown, et al., "Childhood Maltreatment Increases Risk for Personality Disorders During Early Adulthood," *Archives of General Psychiatry* 56 (1999): 600–606.

9. Joel Paris, "Memories of Abuse in Borderline Patients: True or False?" *Harvard Review of Psychiatry* 3 (1995): 10–17.

10. Jane Bybee, Ann Kramer, and Ed Zigler, "Is Repression Adaptive: Relationships to Self-esteem Adjustment, Academic Performance and Self-image," *American Journal of Orthopsychiatry* 67 (1997): 59–59; A. S. Stroebe and W. Stroebe, "Does 'Grief Work' Work?" *Journal of Consulting and Clinical Psychology* 59 (1991): 479–82.

11. Steven M. Southwick, Charles A. Morgan, and Roberta Rosenberg, "Social Sharing of Gulf War Experiences: Association with Trauma-Related Psychological Symptoms," *American Journal of Psychiatry* 188, no. 10 (2000): 703–8; R. Tait and R. C. Silver, "Coming to Terms with Major Negative Life Events," in *Unintended Thoughts,* edited by J. S. Uleman and J. A. Bargh (New York: Guilford Press, 1989), 351–82; J. N. Bohannon, "Flashbulb Memories for the Space Shuttle Disaster: A Tale of Two Theories," *Cognition* (1988): 179–96; C. B. Wortman and R. C. Silver, "The Myths of Coping," *Journal of Personality and Social Psychology* 57 (1991): 349–57.

12. George A. Bonanno, Dachter Kaltner, Are Holen, and Mardi J. Horowitz, "When Avoiding Unpleasant Emotions Might Not Be Such a Bad Thing: Verbal-Autonomic Response Dissociation and Midlife Conjugal Bereavement," *Journal of Personality and Social Psychology* 69, no. 5 (1995): 975–89.

13. E. Foa and D. Riggs, "Post-traumatic Stress Disorder in Rape Victims," *American Psychiatric Press Review of Psychiatry* 12 (1992): 273–303.

14. Bloom, *Creating Sanctuary,* 14.

15. Ann Jennings and Ruth O. Ralph, *In Their Own Words: Trauma Survivors and Professionals They Trust Tell What Hurts, What Helps and What Is Needed for Trauma Services: Maine Trauma Advisory Groups Report 1997* (Augusta: Maine Department of Mental Health Mental Retardation and Substance Abuse Services, June 1997).

16. Ibid., 35, 12, 38.

17. Chrystine Oksana, *Safe Passage to Healing: A Guide for Survivors of Ritual Abuse* (New York: HarperCollins, 1994), 316.

18. Samuel J. Knapp and Leon VandeCreek, *Treating Patients with Memories of Abuse: Legal Risk Management* (Washington, DC: American Psychological Association, 1997), 2.

19. Secret Shame (self-injury information and support), "Self Injury: You Are NOT the Only One," http://www.palace.net/~llama/self-injury/self.html#dbt; accessed April 13, 2000.

20. Bodies Under Siege web-ring, http://www.angelfire.com/or/kharreshome/ busring.html; accessed April 13, 2000.

21. Linda Breslin, personal communication with the author, November 2, 1998.

22. Lynn Williams, "A 'Classic' Case of Borderline Personality Disorder," *Psychiatric Services* 49, no. 2 (1998): 173–74.

23. Marilee Strong, *A Bright Red Scream: Self-Mutilation and the Language of Pain* (New York: Viking, 1998), 57.

24. M. M. Linehan, H. L. Heard, and H. E. Armstrong, "Naturalistic Follow-up of a Behavioral Treatment for Chronically Parasuicidal Borderline Patients," *Archives of General Psychiatry* 50 (1993): 971–74.

25. Peter D. Kramer, "I Contain Multitudes" [review of *Creating Hysteria: Women and Multiple Personality Disorder* by Joan Acocella], *New York Times Book Review,* November 21, 1999.

26. Joan Acocella, "The Politics of Hysteria," *The New Yorker* (April 6, 1998): 64–79, esp. 76.

27. William Anderson, M.D., personal communication with the author, October 17, 1998.

28. Dennis Ratner, Ph.D., personal communication with the author, November 10, 1998.

29. Roger Wilson, M.D., personal communication with the author, November 5, 1998.

30. Dennis R. Fox, "Psychological Jurisprudence and Radical Social Change," *American Psychologist* 48, no. 3 (1993): 234–24, 234. Psychiatry also embraced so-called social and community psychiatry,

especially in the 1960s; see David Musto, "Whatever Happened to Community Psychiatry?" *The Public Interest* (Spring 1975): 53–79. There were several eras of social psychiatry in the twentieth century. The first took place around World War I, the second was after World War II and the third was part of the civil rights era; see E. Fuller Torrey, *Freudian Fraud: The Malignant Effect of Freud's Theory on American Thought and Culture* (New York: HarperCollins, 1992).

31. Laura S. Brown, *Subversive Dialogues: Theory in Feminist Therapy* (New York: Basic Books, 1994), 17.

32. Ibid., 138.

33. K. M. Evans, S. R. Seem, and E. A. Kincade, "Case Approach to Feminist Therapy: A Feminist Therapist's Perspective on Ruth," in *Case Approach to Counseling and Psychotherapy,* edited by G. Corey (Pacific Grove, CA: Brooks/Cole Thomson Learning, 2000), 212–46, 224.

34. Ibid., 229.

35. Feminist Therapy Institute, "The Practice, Politics and Business of Caring: Feminist Approaches to Therapy and Social Change: A Conference for Women in the Allied Mental Health Fields," brochure calling for papers for the Advanced Feminist Therapy Institute 2000 (April 6–9), Portland, Oregon.

36. Feminist Therapy Institute, "Feminist Therapy Ethical Code" (1987).

37. Evans, Seem, and Kincade, "Case Approach to Feminist Therapy," 246.

38. American Psychological Association, "What You Should Know About Women and Depression," www.apa.org/pubinfo/depress.html; accessed April 13, 2000.

39. Ralph W. Heine, "The Negro Patient in Psychotherapy," *Journal of Clinical and Consulting Psychology* 6 (October 1950): 373–76.

40. Elaine Pinderhughes, *Understanding Race, Ethnicity and Power: The Key to Efficacy in Clinical Practice* (New York: Free Press, 1989), 14.

41. American Counseling Association, Counselors for Social Justice, www.counseling.org-/branches_divisions/divisions.htm; accessed April 13, 2000.

42. C. C. Lee and G. R. Walz, eds., *Social Action: A Mandate for Counselors* (Alexandria, VA: American Counseling Association, 1998).

43. Manuel Ramirez III, *Multicultural Psychotherapy: An Approach to Individual and Cultural Differences,* 2nd ed. (Boston: Allyn and Bacon, 1998), 50.

44. Ibid., 48, 49.

45. Patricia Arredondo, Rebecca Toporek, Sherlon Brown, et al., Association for Multicultural Counseling and Development, *Operationalization of the Multicultural Counseling Competencies* (Arlington, VA: American Counseling Association, January 1996), 13, 15.

46. Robbie J. Steward, Robin Powers, Amanda Baden, et al., "Integrating Theory, Research, Training and Practice Toward Multicultural Competency," remarks during the American Counseling Association world conference, Indianapolis, IN, March 28–April 2, 1998; see program guide, March 30, 1998, 45.

47. Morris L. Jackson, Ed.D., personal communication with the author, April 6, 1996.

48. Certification Department, National Board for Certified Counselors, April 7, 2000.

49. Allison Cummings-McCann, remarks during program 358 of the annual meeting of the American Counseling Association, Washington, DC, March 23, 2000.

50. Program 346, 2000 ACA meeting.

51. "Racism: Healing Its Effects," special issue of *Journal of Counseling and Development* 77, no. 1 (1999).

52. Edil Rivera Torres, personal communication with the author, March 28, 2000.

53. Rebecca L. Toporek, "Developing a Common Language and Framework for Understanding Advocacy in Counseling," advocacy paper 14, www.counseling.org/branches_divisions/divisions.htm; accessed April 13, 2000.

54. Derald Wing Sue and David Sue, *Counseling the Culturally Different: Theory and Practice* (New York: John Wiley and Sons, 1990), 6, 207.

55. "Paul," entry in DIVERSEGRAD-@LISTSERVE.AMERICAN.EDU, November 26, 1999.

56. Robert E. Wubbolding, personal communication with the author, December 13, 1999.

57. Sue and Sue, *Counseling the Culturally Different*, 207.

58. Ibid.

59. Freddy A. Paniagua, *Assessing and Treating Culturally Diverse Clients: A Practical Guide* (Thousand Oaks, CA: Sage Publications, 1994), 93. This quotation is taken from tables in the book, which are often naive—in contrast with the text of the book, which is often rich and informative.

60. Ibid., 93.

61. "Regina," list-serve entry, October 14, 1999.

62. C. H. Patterson, "Multicultural Counseling: From Diversity to Universality," *Journal of Counseling and Development* 74 (1996): 227–31, 230.

63. Stephen Weinrach, remarks during a panel presentation, "Alternative Views of Multicultural Counseling," program 281, 2000 ACA meeting.

64. Program 135, 2000 ACA meeting.

65. Program 157, 2000 ACA meeting.

66. "Chris," list-serve entry, March 30, 2000.

67. Clemmont Vontress, personal communication with the author, March 31, 2000.

68. Program 490, 2000 ACA meeting.

69. American Counseling Association, proposal preparation guidelines for 2000 Learning Institutes.

70. American Counseling Association, evaluation form for 2000 Learning Institutes.

71. Stephen G. Weinrach and Kenneth R. Thomas, "Diversity-Sensitive Counseling Today: A Postmodern Clash of Values," *Journal of Counseling and Development* 76 (1998): 115–22.

72. Center for Substance Abuse Prevention, *An African-Centered Model of Prevention for African-American Youth at High Risk*, technical report 6 (Rockville, MD: U.S. Department of Health and Human Services, 1993).

73. Leonard C. Long, *An Afrocentric Intervention Strategy*, technical report 6 (Rockville, MD: U.S. Department of Health and Human Services, 1993), 87–92, esp. 90.

74. Lauretta Omeltschenko, personal communication with the author, January 9, 2000.

75. American Counseling Association, "Code of Ethics and Standards of Practice" (1997), A5b, A6a.

76. Brian Canfield, personal communication, March 31, 2000.

77. Clemmont Vontress, personal communication with the author, March 31, 2000.

78. Alan Charles Kors, "Thought Reform 101," *Reason* (March 2000): 26–34, 26.

79. "Kelley," list-serve entry, December 5, 1999.

80. "Chicago Agencies to Launch Nation's First Psychotherapist Certificate Program for Working with Les/Bi/Gay/Trans Clients," *MedscapeWire* (January 13, 2000).

81. Quoted in "Counseling Today Online" (December 1998), http:www.couseling.org/members/ctonline/ct1298/conversion_therapy.cfm.

82. American Counseling Association, "Counselors Say Conversion Therapy Claims Are Groundless and Prejudicial," http://www.counseling.org/search/SearchAction.cfm.

83. American Psychological Association, "Psychology in Daily Life: Answers to Your Questions About Sexual Orientation and Homosexuality," http://helping.apa.org/daily/answers.html#cantherapychange; accessed April 13, 2000.

84. "APA Maintains Reparative Therapy Not Effective," press release, January 15, 1999, http://www.psycho.org/psycho/htdocs/pnews/99-01-15/therapy.html.

85. National Association of Social Workers, "Policy Statement: Lesbian, Gay and Bisexual Issues," approved by delegate assembly, August 1996; reprinted in *Social Work Speaks*, 4th ed. (Washington, DC: National Association of Social Workers Press, 1997).

86. Mark D. Schiller, M.D., personal communication with the author, April 5, 1996; Douglas Tucker, M.D., personal communication with the author, April 12, 2000.

87. Susan D. Scheidt, "Great Expectations: Challenges for Women as Mental Health Administrators," *Journal of Mental Health Administration* 21, no. 4 (1994): 419–29.

88. Department of Public Health, City and County of San Francisco, "Experience Criteria Utilized for Certification for African American Health Services Specialist" (1996).

89. Michelle Clark, "The UCSF/San Francisco General Hospital's Black Focus Inpatient Service: A Decade of Experience," remarks at the annual meeting of the American Psychiatric Association, New York, May 7, 1996.

90. Alvin F. Poussaint, "They Hate. They Kill. Are They Insane?" *New York Times,* August 26, 1999.

91. Emily Eakin, "Bigotry as a Mental Illness or Just Another Norm?" *New York Times,* January 15, 2000.

92. Robert L. Spitzer, "Racism Is Not a Treatable Illness" (letter to the editor), *New York Times,* August 30, 1999.

93. Charles Krauthammer, "Screwball Psychologizing," *Washington Post,* January 14, 2000.

Index

About the Author

S ALLY SATEL, M.D., A PRACTICING PSYCHIATRIST, is a lecturer at Yale University School of Medicine and the W. H. Brady Fellow at the American Enterpise Institute. Her articles have appeared in *The New Republic,* the *Wall Street Journal,* and the *New York Times,* and she is a frequent contributor to medical journals. She lives in Washington, D.C.